DIABETICS and DIET

Published by :
Lotus Press Publishers & Distributors

DIABETICS and DIET

Vijaya Kumar

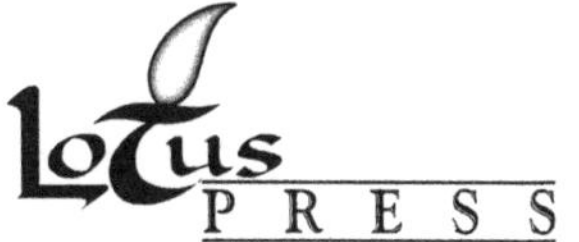

4735/22, Prakash Deep Building
Ansari Road, Darya Ganj,
New Delhi - 110002

Lotus Press : Publishers & Distributors
Unit No. 220, 2nd Floor, 4735/22, Prakash Deep Building,
Ansari Road, Darya Ganj, New Delhi- 110002
Ph.: 41325510, 98118-38000
• E-mail : lotuspress1984@gmail.com
www.lotuspress.co.in

Diabetics and Diet

ISBN: 81-901912-6-9

Printed & Published by : **Lotus Press Publishers & Distributors,** New Delhi-02

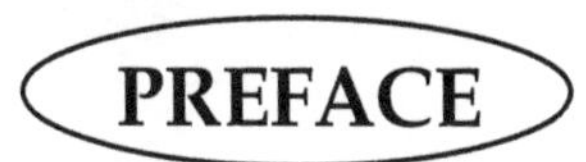

PREFACE

Diabetes is a nutritional disorder. Though it is related to sugar, but it depends on overall intake of food. Whatever we eat, it is converted into blood glucose, which provides energy to our body. But when this blood glucose is not digested/absorbed properly due to any reason, the level of sugar increases and becomes diabetes.

The persons who arc obese, are more at risk of diabetes. This disease, if not treated properly, causes dullness, lethargy, loss of weight etc. In severe conditions, it affects kidneys, heart, eyes and nerves also.

This book contains a detailed information of each and every aspect of this disease. It's types, causes, symptoms, prevention and treatment is elaborated properly, including insulin injections etc; for the benefit of readers. There are separate chapters for diet and exercise.

The care of feet, eyes and heart is also discussed separately besides the proper diet plan and exercises for the diabetics.

India is also emerging as a country of diabetics, as the ratio of sufferers of this disease is increasing day-by-day.

Hope readers will be benefitted by this book.

—Author

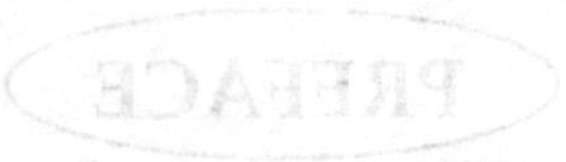

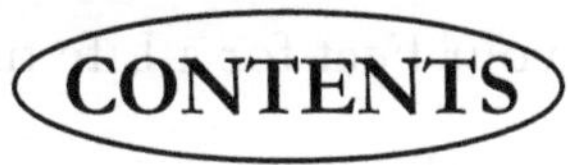

CONTENTS

1

INTRODUCTION AND TYPES OF DIABETES

Diabetes was once regarded as one of the more serious diseases, but today it is easily controlled and managed. A patient's participation in the treatment goes a long way in averting long-term complications, and hence has a significant impact on a better quality of life. Physiological control and good health are essential in altering the progression of this disease.

Unlike other diseases, diabetes involves your entire body, from your body organ systems to the mind. Controlling your diabetes on day-to-day basis can require a lot of self-discipline. Those who have lived life fully with the fullest complications and the best control have been those who have focused their active lifestyles around good health habits and dietary control as well as proper insulin therapy, and a general reduction of high risk factors for disease. Planning for good health involves continuing education in your disease.

What is Diabetes?

Diabetes is a disease that sets in due to the body's inability to make proper use of the foods consumed as a result of insufficient insulin. Bacteria, viruses or other microbes do not cause it. Due to the inability on the part of the body to perform certain vital functions, the diabetic is unable to use the carbohydrates, the sugars and starches, and convert them into heat and energy that his body needs to operate normally.

The carbohydrates that you eat are converted into a form of sugar known as glucose, which the cells in the body use as a source of energy. This glucose increases the level of blood glucose, which in turn helps in the release of a hormone known as insulin. This insulin is released from the islet cells of the pancreas, a gland in the abdomen, and the level of glucose in the blood is regulated by insulin which assists in utilising and storing glucose in the body.

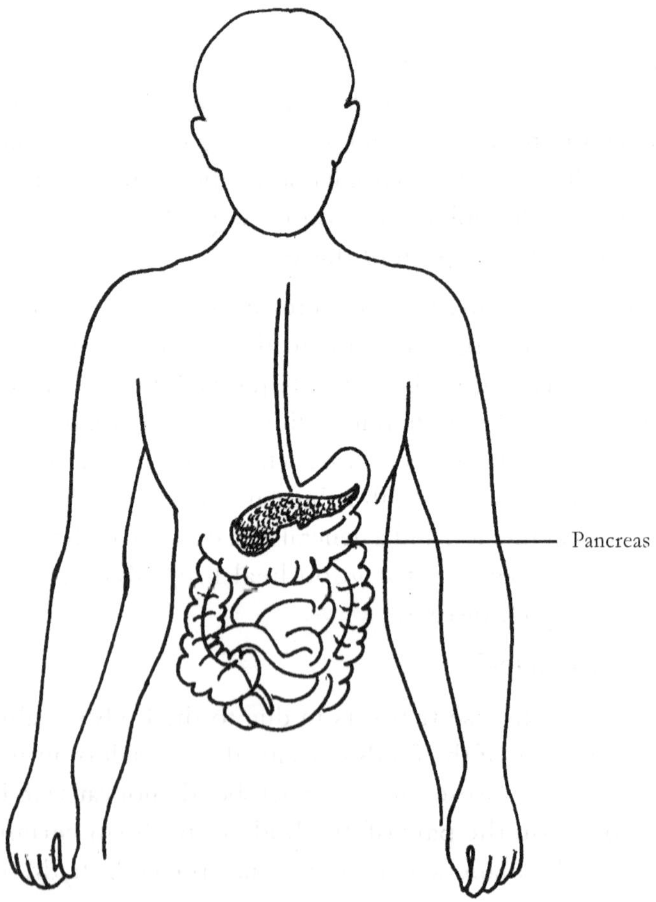

The body needs insulin, and most people have sufficient supply of it. A diabetic may have none at all, or probably not sufficient to aid in the transfer of the glucose from the blood to the respective cells. When there is no insulin, glucose builds up in the body, leading to diabetes.

Though there is no cure for diabetes, yet it can be controlled. It is not contagious. A diabetic should know everything about the disease – its nature, problems, treatment, control, self-help remedies, etc. Armed with these facts, he will be better equipped to cope with the disease every day of his life.

The body to make possible all the numerous physical and chemical activities necessary for life uses the nutrients that we consume and the oxygen that we breathe in. Metabolism involves two processes known as anabolism and catabolism. Anabolism means building up, while catabolism means breaking down.

The food that we eat is reduced by digestion into simple chemicals. These are rearranged and built into new cells, tissues, blood, bone, muscles, etc. Cells and tissues that have served their purpose, and are no longer in use, are broken down into simple chemicals. They may either be eliminated as waste from the body, or rearranged and used in some other form. During this process, energy is released.

To maintain good health, there is need for a balance between the foods we eat and the metabolic requirements of the body. Starvation leads to depletion of energy and chemicals, while excess food leads to storage of fat in the body, and hence obesity.

With age the metabolic activity slows down, and a diabetic shows symptoms of starvation. While a starved person can assimilate the carbohydrates that he eats, the diabetic has them but cannot use them. The unused glucose amasses in the bloodstream and tissues, and the excess gets into the urine. The kidneys strain to eliminate the excess sugar, causing water also to be eliminated. Dehydration with insatiable thirst sets in.

When the body is starved of energy, it begins to consume itself, leading to the formation of poisonous chemicals known as ketone bodies. Gradually acidosis sets in, and, if neglected, it leads to coma, and finally death.

TYPES OF DIABETES

Diabetes exists in many different forms. There are two groups, which are mainly recognised.

Diabetics below 40 years of age generally have the disease setting in, in a fairly dramatic way. They always need insulin injections. About 30 per cent of all diabetics fall into this category, known as Insulin Dependent Diabetes, or IDD or Type I.

Older persons develop diabetes with less obvious symptoms and may be often overweight. This group is not dependent on insulin injections, and is known as the non-Insulin Dependent Diabetes, or INDD or Type II. There are exceptions to both cases though.

Diabetes Mellitus

Commonly called simply diabetes, this is a disorder in which the body is unable to control the sugar as a source of energy.

When carbohydrate foods containing sugar and starch are digested, they are absorbed into the bloodstream as glucose. Insulin is released into the bloodstream when the level of glucose rises, and the hormone enables glucose to be stored and used in tissues. In diabetes, there is insufficient insulin, and in severe cases, there is no insulin at all.

Long-term complications may be caused by abnormalities in the structure of blood vessels, which can affect the eyes, kidneys, heart and legs. Early treatment prevents or delays these developments.

Diabetes Insipidus

This rare disease has nothing in common with diabetes mellitus, except the persistent passing of large volumes of urine and constant thirst. It is caused by a disturbance of a secretion of the pituitary gland, vasopressin, which controls the rate at which water is eliminated from the kidneys.

Impaired Glucose Tolerance

This refers to the condition is which fasting plasma glucose level is normal, but after glucose intake, the levels are abnormally elevated.

Gestational Diabetes

This refers to diabetes that develops during pregnancy. In the majority of cases, glucose tolerance will return to normal after delivery.

2

SYMPTOMS AND CAUSES OF DIABETES

Thirst

The first signs of diabetes, especially in a young person, are thirst and loss of weight, both interrelated. The continual loss of fluid from the body dries it out; feeling thirsty is a warning that unless they drink enough to replace the extra urine that is eliminated they will soon be in trouble.

The resulting thirst is usually mild in the early stages, and most people do not realise its significance unless someone else has diabetes. Someone with undiagnosed diabetes may wake up at night to quench his thirst and frequently urinate, and still not realise that something is wrong.

Frequent Urination

The first thing to go wrong in a diabetic is increased amount of urine. Normally, a person passes about one and a half litres of urine per day, but someone who has uncontrolled diabetes may produce five times that amount. This leads to dehydration and excessive thirst; of course, people without diabetes too may pass large amounts of urine. Beer drinkers know this to be true!

Weight Loss

In spite of a healthy appetite, there is weight loss. Glucose that is obtained from the digestion of sugary or starchy food accumulates in the body of a diabetic. It overflows into the urine, and body tissues get broken down to form glucose and ketones, which causes weight loss. Someone with uncontrolled diabetes may lose as much as 1,000 grammes of glucose in their urine in a day, leading to weight loss.

Exhaustion

A feeling of sheer exhaustion or weakness may result in the person's inability to cope with the daily routine.

Itching and Soreness around Genitals

Itching or redness around her vagina and inner thighs may trouble a woman whose diabetes is out of control. Men may also experience soreness around the end of their penis. If the foreskin is also affected, it may become thickened, thus preventing the foreskin from being pulled back, and making it impossible to keep the penis clean.

If you keep your urine free from glucose by controlling the diabetes, the itching and soreness will normally clear up. An anti-yeast cream may speed up the improvement while the glucose is cleared from the urine.

Blurred Vision

A diabetic may have blurred vision due to the damage of the retina at the back of the eye. Since the minor changes in the retina take years to develop, they are never seen early on in the disease in younger people. In some case, in older people, the retina may already be damaged by the time the diabetes is discovered.

The lens of the eye can also be affected in diabetes. The blurred vision can be corrected by wearing glasses. When the disease is out of control, the lens of the eye becomes swollen, resulting in short sight. The lens returns to its normal shape once the diabetes is under control.

Boils and Carbuncles

Often diabetes is detected because of boils. The skin and the underlying tissue may become hard, red and sensitive with pus oozing out at several points. This often occurs on the back and nape of the neck.

CAUSES

The main cause is that the body is unable to produce enough insulin for the body's needs. Why this is so is not so well understood. A few clues do give a lead to the causes.

Diabetes may run in families, being hereditary. A child of a non-diabetic can become diabetic, since the disease may skip generations because of genetic coding that prevents it from appearing in every generation.

If a person has a tendency to develop diabetes, then obesity may bring on the disease. This mostly occurs in middle-aged or older people. In most cases, diabetes can be controlled by dieting and weight loss. Many obese people with diabetes find it difficult to shed off the excess weight, while others find they have to supplement strict dieting with tablets or insulin injections.

If a mother has diabetes during pregnancy but recovers soon after her baby is born she does carry a slightly increased risk of diabetes for the rest of her life. The baby does not carry this risk.

Who Gets Diabetes?

Practically, anyone can get diabetes, regardless of age, sex, race, place, etc. There are increasing numbers of diabetics reported every year. One out of every four diabetics gets the disease before he turns 50 years of age. There are numerous cases of the disease in childhood, adolescence and young adulthood.

All of us are susceptible to diabetes throughout our lifetimes. The susceptibility generally subsides at 80 years and thereafter.

Females are more susceptible to the disease. At the age of 30 years, a woman becomes more susceptible until, between 45 and 65 years, she is twice as likely as a man to get the disease. As she approaches menopause, a striking rise in susceptibility occurs.

The highest number of deaths from diabetes is among single women, being almost twice as great as among single women. The death rate from diabetes among married men is lower than that of bachelors, widowers or divorcees. A woman with more children is more susceptible to the disease than a woman with fewer children. The more pregnancies a woman undergoes, the greater is the possibility that she will become diabetic.

Obese people are also prone to develop diabetes. Those who eat more are susceptible to diabetes than those who eat a limited quantity. The greater the food intake, and the lesser the metabolic need, the greater the possibility of developing diabetes. A popular misconception is that healthy people who eat sweets are prone to get diabetes. This is not true. Some of the countries have lower diabetes records though they have the highest sugar consumption.

When a person eats more than he should, the pancreas has to produce extra insulin to handle the carbohydrates. The body generally copes with this extra demand for insulin, but if the process continues, production of insulin drops, and insulin deficiency results. This leads to diabetes. Since this exists only due to abnormal eating, reduction of food intake and weight can restore the metabolic balance and control the diabetes.

Heredity influence is often a very elusive factor. A diabetic may very healthy parents and grandparents without diabetes, but that still does not eliminate the possibility of a hereditary predisposition.

When diabetes appears in a family, it seems to develop earlier in each succeeding generation – the second generation gets it earlier than the first, the third gets it even earlier than the second, and so on.

A person with disturbances of the endocrine glands may develop diabetes. Liver disease can bring on diabetes by affecting the body's sugar balance. People with overactive thyroid glands and the frontal lobe of the pituitary gland seem to be susceptible to the disease.

3

TREATMENT WITHOUT INSULIN

Diet

In younger people, there is need to start insulin injections fairly soon, but in older people with diabetes, the disease can be controlled without insulin, unless they are terribly ill. They are usually advised to change the type and quantity of food that they eat, especially in overweight people. If change of diet does not bring about the diabetes control, then tablets are normally tried first by adding them to the diet. If these do not work then insulin is the only alternative.

It is very important to know about the right type of ford and the quantity that you eat. People who develop diabetes later in life are often overweight. They can normally do without insulin injections, and follow a good diet and take certain tablets. Achieving and maintaining a sensible weight therefore helps you to improve your control of diabetes. It also helps in reducing other health hazards related with obesity, like high blood pressure and heart ailments.

Ideally, your calorie intake from the food you consume should balance the amount of energy used by your body. This will help you in maintaining your weight. If the quantity of food and drink you take provides more calories than normally taken, then the extra food will be converted into body fat and you will put on weight. An obese person therefore needs to cut down on the calories, so that you take less energy than your body needs. Your body will make up the difference by using up the fat stored in your body, and you will subsequently lose weight.

Those on medication for diabetes are usually advised to keep fairly close to regular meal times to avoid getting a low blood sugar (hypo). A person whose diabetes is controlled by diet alone has very little risk of hypo, and hence he need not keep to strict meal times. It is however easier to control diabetes if you have three or so small meals a day rather than one or two large ones.

Once you have developed diabetes, it will remain with you forever. By adhering strictly to the food plan, your diabetes can be well controlled.

Snacking in between meals is generally recommended only for insulin-dependent diabetics to balance the effect of the insulin they take. For non-insulin dependents, too may snacks can cause a problem of weight gain!

A caution for those who love to linger on food, and are diabetic – do not eat as many diabetic foods as you like. They are no lower in fats or calories than ordinary food. They only replace ordinary sugar with a substitute.

The only special foods recommended for diabetics are the ones labelled as 'diet' or 'low calorie'. These are marketed for people wishing to keep their weight under control.

Weight

People who are of normal weight during the time of diagnosis are more likely to need treatment with insulin or tablets rather than with just diet. If you are overweight, by losing just 3 kilogrammes is enough to restore the blood glucose to normal, while in another person the blood glucose remains high even after losing several kilogrammes. It is better to remain slim rather then be obese.

For an overweight person, a loss of half to one kilogramme of weight a week is good. Losing weight slowly and steadily is the healthiest way. Most people can manage to shed off weight simply by modifying the quantities and types of food they eat, especially by cutting down the quantities of fats, sugar and alcohol they consume.

Though some people eat very little, yet they find it difficult to lose weight, while another person may be eating four times more and yet remain slim. This is due to the metabolic rate at which the food is burnt up. Those who burn up their food fast, remain slim.

The only way a person with a sluggish metabolic rate can lose weight is by eating less food than the body requires, so that, he burns up the stores of fat in his body. To lose weight, you need to concentrate on reducing the amount of fat you eat, and cut down on foods that contain both fat and sugar, especially biscuits and confectionery. Also by increasing the amount of regular exercise, you can help activate the metabolic rate at which you burn up food.

Tablets

These are only effective when a reasonable amount of natural insulin is produced. They should always be used along with a diet that restricts sugary foods. In elderly, overweight people, the first line of treatment is generally diet, and tablets should be used only when absolutely necessary.

The two most commonly used groups of tablets prescribed for diabetics are the sulphonylureas and biguanides. The former includes chlorpropamide, glibenclamide, gliclazide, glipizide, gliquidone and tolbutamide, whereas the latter includes metformin.

The two most commonly used tablets, glibenclamide and chlorpropamide, belong to the same group, sulphonylureas. The former tablet acts for about 19 hours, and is taken once or twice a day. The latter acts for 36 hours and hence needs to be restricted to one a day. In the elderly people, the long action of chlorpropamide may leave the person with a very low blood glucose level for several days, and hence care has to be taken while prescribing it.

Metformin can cause a curious taste in the mouth. It can be substituted with other tablets like glibenclamide or chlorpropamide.

Non-Medical Treatments

Complementary therapies can be tried alongside conventional medicine. Yoga, reflexology, aromatherapy, etc., can benefit someone with diabetes to feel more relaxed. As stress can have a detrimental effect on blood glucose control, it may mean that diabetes improves as a result.

These therapies should always be complementary to your usual diabetes treatment. Many plants are said to reduce the high level of flood glucose in diabetics. A berry from West Africa and the bittergourd have some effect on lowering blood glucose, but these can be taken along with the conventional tablets which are more convenient, more reliable and safer. Herbal remedies have no effect on insulin-dependent diabetics.

4

TREATMENT WITH INSULIN

Insulin may be needed at any age but is generally essential in young people. The discovery of the hormone is 1921 by Frederick Banting and Charlie's Best in Toronto revolutionised the outlook of millions of diabetics. Long-acting and short-acting forms of insulin are made, which are given as one or two injections each day. The choice of insulin depends on the individual patient's requirements.

One-third of the diabetics need insulin. Insulin overaction, or more rarely reaction to sulphonylureas, may cause too great a fall of the blood sugar level (hypoglycaemia). The early symptoms are weakness, trembling, sweating, hunger and tingling around the mouth. Double vision, mental confusion and drowsiness follow and eventually consciousness may be lost. Other possible causes are a delay between meals (so that the injected insulin is not used up) or excessive exercise.

Treatment of hypoglycaemia is to eat two or three lumps or spoons of sugar immediately after the symptoms are recognised. All diabetics on insulin should carry sugar, as well as an identification card stating their treatment and measures to be taken for an insulin reaction.

Insulin has to be injected as it is inactivated when taken orally. Virtually all those who develop diabetics when young need insulin from the time of diagnosis. The elderly may manage without it for several years on other forms of treatment, but eventually many of them will need insulin to supplement their diminishing supply from their pancreas.

The short-acting insulin is injected under the skin, and this lasts for about six hours. Nowadays, many people who need insulin have a combination of short and long acting insulin, twice a day, and several have insulin four times a day with an insulin pen.

Many people have been using pork or beef insulin, but nowadays human insulin is on the rise. It is either made from bacteria to produce insulin that has the same structure as human insulin, or from pork insulin modified to resemble human insulin. It is rigorously purified and cannot be a source of injection.

It is best to have your insulin half an hour before a meal. It is judicious to keep your two injections, if you need two, approximately 12 hours apart.

Good control of diabetes depends not just on the dose of insulin, but the site you choose for your injections (upper arms, abdomen, buttocks, thighs), the timing and type of food you eat, and the amount of exercise you take.

Diet and Insulin

When a person starts on insulin after years of strict diet and tablets, he may have to change his diet by restricting the amount of carbohydrates he eats.

Everyone with diabetes needs a food plan to help the balance of food eaten against the amount of insulin and exercise taken. The simplest plan just encourages you to eat some carbohydrate foods at each meal. A more detailed plan would tell you about the amounts of proteins and fats you should eat. Fats should be taken is small quantities as excess of it can lead to overweight problems. The aim of your food plan is to eat approximately the same quantities of carbohydrate and calories at much the same time every day.

Nowadays, we realise that it is not just the number of exchanges that matter. Different foods affect blood glucose levels in different ways even when their carbohydrate content is the same. It is the total calories you eat that affects whether or not you are overweight, and that a fibre-rich diet is good for all. The type and quality of carbohydrates rich in fibre usually take longer to digest, do not raise the blood glucose quite so much or so quickly, and keep the blood glucose at a steady level for longer, which helps to prevent hypos. They all consist of more vitamins and minerals, and are believed to prevent the build-up of excess fat in the arteries.

If you are on two insulin injections per day, never skip even a single one as the blood glucose level will rise even if you have no carbohydrates.

People taking insulin sometimes need to eat snacks in between meals. When the pancreas functions normally, it produces insulin when you eat, and 'switches off' when the food has been used up. Insulin that has been injected does not 'switch off' in this way. Since it has a peak effect at certain times of the day it is important to cover its action by eating a certain number of carbohydrates, or you will have a hypo. The carbohydrate rich in fibre will last longer as it is then more slowly absorbed.

Injection Technique

Do not use spirit before or after injecting yourself, as it tends to harden the skin. If you must clean the injection site, use soap and water only.

Ensure that very large quantities of air is not injected directly into the circulation, as this could be dangerous and produce an airlock in the bloodstream. Tiny air bubbles would not do any harm, and would quickly be absorbed.

When you have to use two types of insulin, and mix them in the same syringe, draw up the clear (short-acting) insulin first followed by the cloudy (long-acting) insulin, to prevent the clear syringe becoming cloudy.

Insulin has to be injected into the deep layer of fat under the skin, but not into the muscle. It is advisable to first pinch up a generous amount of skin, without squeezing too tightly, and then pushes the needle in quickly at right angles to the skin. If the needle is pushed through the skin quickly, the injection should be virtually painless.

Sometimes, after giving yourself insulin injection you may notice slight bleeding. This is due to the puncture of a blood capillary, but you need not worry; just press quickly with your finger or tissue over the site to stop the bleeding.

Insulin sometimes leaks out immediately after an injection. At such times, move the skin to one side immediately after removing the syringe, or do this before inserting the needle in the skin. If these fail, then press straight on the spot after the injection.

Injection Sites

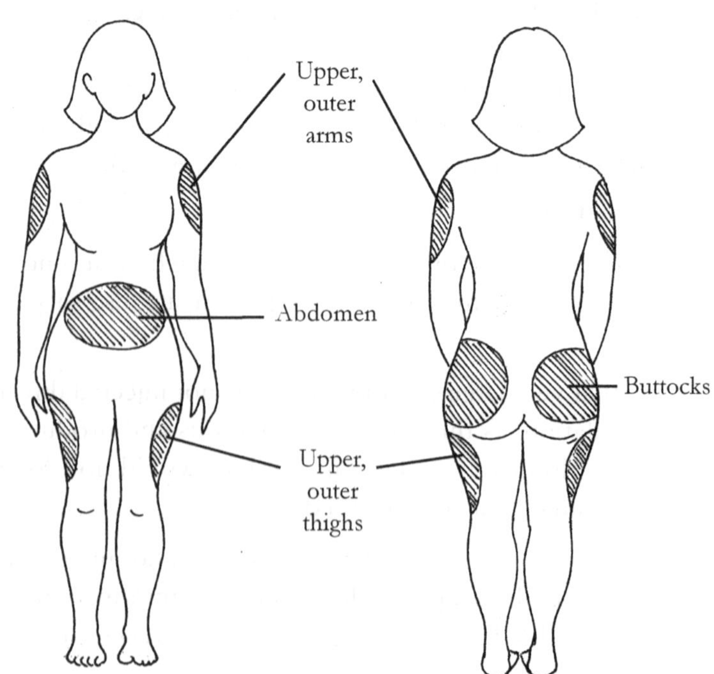

Insulin should be given into the deep layers of fat below the skin, anywhere in the body where there is a reasonable layer of fat. The best places are the front and side of middle or upper thighs, upper and outer arms, buttocks and the abdomen. It is very important to change to new sites regularly to prevent unsightly lumps.

Insulin is absorbed at different rates from different areas of the body. The abdomen and arms are the sites for the fastest rate of absorption, while the thighs and buttocks are the sites for the slowest absorption. Insulin is more quickly absorbed from the thighs and buttocks if you exercise soon after the injection. Insulin absorption is also faster after a hot bath or sunbathing.

Insulin Pens

An insulin pen has a cartridge of insulin inside a fountain pen-like case, which is used with a special disposable needle, which is finely coated with silicon. After dialling the required number of units of insulin, a button is pressed, and the pen releases the correct dose of insulin. Only one type of insulin can be injected with this pen at a time.

The great advantage of the pen is that you need not carry syringes and bottles of insulin. Especially for people with arthritis in the hands, the dial-a-dose clicking action is easier to use than drawing up insulin in a conventional syringe.

Pumps and Injectors

Insulin pumps consist of a slow motor driving a syringe containing insulin, which is pumped down a fine bore tube and needle. The needle is inserted under the skin and strapped in place. There is also a device to give meal time boosts of insulin.

Insulin pump has benefited many people in successfully controlling their blood glucose. With the introduction of insulin pens, these pumps are becoming less popular.

The main problem with pumps is that like all machines they are capable of going wrong. If the pump suddenly stops, the user will quickly go into a state of complete insulin starvation, and may quickly develop ketoacidosis. Since the needle remains under the skin, it acts as a foreign body, and may lead to an infected abscess. Furthermore, the pump has to be worn day and night, and so becomes a constant reminder of the diabetes.

Insulin Administration

1. It is always best to use disposable syringe and needle. If not, they must be sterilised in boiling soft water for at least five minutes.
2. Ensure that the insulin in the vial is well mixed, by shaking the vial well before use.
3. Make sure that the syringe is totally free of any water.
4. Wash the site for injection with soap and water.
5. Wipe the rubber stopper in the vial with a piece of cotton wet with alcohol. Never remove the stopper.
6. Set the plunger of your syringe at the mark showing your dose.
7. Insert the needle through the rubber stopper of the vial, and push the plunger all the way in. This forces air into the vial.

8. Turn the vial slowly upside down several times. Then, with the vial upside down, pull the plunger back to the mark showing your dose.
9. Stick the needle into the injection site quickly and deeply with the needle going straight in, not at an angle. Push the plunger in slowly as far as it will go.
10. Hold the cotton piece lightly over the spot where the needle enters the skin. Then pull out the needle, continuing to hold the cotton on the skin for a few seconds, just press, but do not rub the spot.
11. If disposable, then throw away the syringe and the needle, or else, to reuse later on, wash the syringe with clear water and return it to the tube.

Insulin Equipment

1. *Insulin:* The patient should always stock extra vials of insulin in a cool place in case of emergency such as coma or acidosis.
2. *Syringe:* The syringe used should be matched to the strength of the insulin; this will prevent errors in dosage. It could be either of glass or plastic. In India, the disposable insulin syringe commonly available is of 1 ml capacity, with U40 or U100 embossed on its barrel.

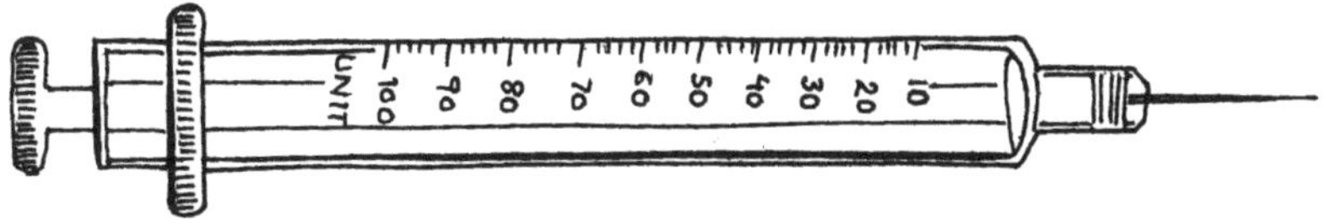

3. *Hypodermic Needle:* The needle should be of stainless steel, ½ to 5/8 inch long, with a 25 to 26 gauge. You should always store a reserve supply of needles, for they may bend or break.

4. *Sterile Case:* This is needed to keep the syringe and needle at home or for travel. This case should also be sterilised.

5. *Alcohol and Sterile Cotton:* These are needed for sterilisation of the top of the insulin vial and the cotton to be placed on the injected spot while the needle is being taken out of the skin.

5

BLOOD GLUCOSE TESTS

One can live a successful life by achieving good blood glucose control. The degree of success can be measured only by measurements of the body's response to treatment. If you are a diabetic and you feel well, it does not mean that you are well controlled. It is only when control goes wrong that you wake up to the fact the something is wrong. Too low blood glucose may show symptoms of hypo, and excess glucose will show symptoms of excess thirst, frequent urination, weakness and fatigue. Many different tests allow precise measurement of control.

Blood Glucose Tests

For a normal person, the blood glucose before meals ranges from 65 mg to 110 mg, and after meals it may rise as high as 180 mg, depending on the carbohydrate content of his meal. Even when he starves, his blood glucose concentration never drops below 65 mg, and however much he eats, it never goes above 180 mg.

In the past few years, diabetic patients have been encouraged to do their own glucose measurements. It is suited for both insulin treated as well as tablets and diet following people.

It is important to keep the bottle of sticks for blood glucose monitoring dry and kept in a cool place.

When glucose is given to a normal person, his blood glucose level does rise following its absorption into the blood. But various mechanisms act to keep the blood glucose levels within normal limits. This is called normal tolerance to glucose or normal glucose tolerance. When the blood glucose levels rise above certain set limits after a standard glucose intake, the person is said to have diabetes mellitus.

The easiest and fastest process for measuring glucose and ketones in the blood is to use plastic or paper strips like those used in urine tests. These strips give a range, not an exact value. Reagent kits and rapid analytical systems are other methods to test blood glucose. These tests use chemicals to test blood samples in a rapid single-step process.

Blood sugar is affected by the food eaten, the amount of time after or before eating, and activity and stress. A sample taken within two hours after you have eaten gives the most sensitive results after a measured glucose intake. The fasting glucose concentration is the measure of blood sugar after a lack of intake for more than four hours or overnight. If you have diabetes, your glucose concentration is usually the lowest in this state.

It is usually easiest to obtain blood from the fingertips. The sides of the fingertips are less sensitive than the fleshy part of the fingertips.

Urine Tests

Urine tests are basic diagnostic tools that can give physicians valuable information about how your body is working.

In the semi-quantitative urine testing method, the physician may use either a tablet or paper or plastic strips to determine the approximate sugar or ketone level in your urine. A small sample of urine is sufficient, and the test takes just a few seconds. The strips coated with chemicals change colour according to sugar and ketone concentration. For example, one type of string has colour ranging from yellow through green to dark blue. With this test, a colour that is close to dark blue indicates a high concentration of sugar in the urine. However, certain medications like vitamin C, aspirin, etc., may interfere with the colours on the strip and give distorted readings.

The disadvantage of urine tests, in general, is that they are less accurate and more difficult to interpret than blood tests. This is because the point at which your kidneys begin to spill glucose into your urine may differ from the point in other people.

In the quantitative measurement method, only glucose and ketones are measured, and the other chemicals in your blood responsible for distorted readings are removed. Another advantage is that the exact concentration, instead of a range, of glucose and ketones in the urine is measured.

In urine testing, if the physician asks for a 24-hour urine sample, this means that all the urine during that period must be collected and taken to the laboratory.

Urine in the kidneys is formed by filtration of blood. When the glucose concentration in the blood is below 180 mg, any glucose filtered into the urine is subsequently reabsorbed into the body. When it exceeds that limit, more glucose is filtered than the body can absorb and it passes in the urine. In this condition the amount of glucose in the urine will be in proportion to the level of glucose in the blood.

Ketones are breakdown products of the fat stored in the body, and present in small amounts in all people. They are dangerous only in large amounts, and diabetic patients have to be very careful to check an excess of it. The symptoms are excessive thirst, passing large amounts of urine, and nausea.

Usually, if glucose and ketones appear together, it indicates poor diabetes control, although this may be a passing phase, with their disappearance by noon. If they persist all the time, then you do need to improve your control of diabetes.

The first test in the morning before breakfast is ideal. If it is continually negative, try occasionally before lunch, or before evening meal, or at bedtime. If these are all negative, you can try two or three hours after breakfast when you are most likely to find glucose in the urine.

GLYCOSYLATED HAEMOGLOBIN (GHb or GHbA1)

Glycosylated haemoglobin is the combination of haemoglobin (Hb) and glucose (G). The red blood cells are bathed in plasma that contains glucose. Glucose gets attached to haemoglobin in an irreversible fashion to form GHb. Glycosylated haemoglobin testing gives a more accurate idea of the long-term control of diabetes.

The concentration of these glycosylated haemoglobin molecules is a good barometer of average glucose content, as it is higher in diabetics than in non-diabetics, and very high in patients who have poor control over their diabetes.

Since the lifespan of red blood cells is about four months, a high concentration of glycolated haemoglobin in your blood is a sign that the condition has been building up over a period of time. The measurement of glycosylated haemoglobin gives an indication of what happened previously, rather than what is taking place now. This helps the physician to establish or make adjustments in your treatments. The tests are useful for long-term monitoring diabetic control, considering the fact that they are expensive.

Glucose Tolerance Test

This test measures the ability of a person to handle a standard amount of glucose. The glucose is usually given orally. The test involves taking a small specimen of blood from a vein in your arm. Over several hour periods, multiple separate readings of blood glucose are taken. These measurements, plotted on a graph, graphically show how your body handles glucose. The test is especially valuable as it can confirm the presence of a condition called impaired glucose tolerance.

Those with impaired glucose tolerance do have high blood glucose levels after meals, but this may not necessarily be diabetes as their fasting sugar is normal. However, such people are more likely than others to develop active diabetes.

In a normal person, the fasting blood glucose level is between 65 and 100 mg per ml of blood. After taking glucose solution, it rises within half an hour or so, but does not exceed 150 mg per ml of blood. The blood glucose returns to the fasting level within two hours. Glucose does not get spilled in urine at any stage.

Glucose Concentration Value (mg per ml of blood)

Normal

1.	Fasting value	65-100
2.	2 hours after meals	100-120

Impaired Glucose Tolerance

1.	Fasting value	105-120
2.	2 hours after glucose intake	120-150

Diabetes Mellitus

1.	Fasting value	> 120
2.	2 hours after glucose intake	> 180

A glucose tolerance test is usually done in the morning after three days of good eating so that your body can handle sugar optimally. The first test is done before breakfast so that it will reflect your fasting glucose to be taken orally. On very rare occasions glucose is taken intravenously. At various hourly intervals after glucose consumption, blood samples will be taken to measure the glucose level.

Impaired glucose tolerance is the term used instead of borderline, chemical or latent diabetes. Patients with such tolerance may have to undergo other tests.

Steroid Glucose Tolerance Test

This is a variation of the glucose tolerance test. A steroid (cortisma) that mimics stress in the body is given to the patient. If this test shows impaired glucose tolerance, then it is a warning that he may develop diabetes, especially if other members in his family have it.

6

PLANNING A DIABETIC DIET

Diet constitutes an essential part of treatment of diabetes. Many obese diabetics can be treated by diet alone. Those on insulin or tablets have to follow a strict standard diet. In the treatment of diabetes, there is no substitute for diet.

Planning a Diet

The first step in planning a diet is to determine the calorie allowance. This depends on the age, activities, physiological needs, sex, etc. A diabetic doing manual work needs more calories than a sedentary diabetic.

An overweight diabetic needs to lose excess weight, and hence a diet providing 1,000-1,200 kcals is enough for him. A sedentary diabetic of overage weight needs a diet of 1,700-1,800 kcals. A diabetic housewife with light work requires around 1,600 kcals. Young diabetics, losing weight on developing diabetes, need a diet of 2,500 kcals or more. A labourer who is a diabetic may require a diet having 3,000 kcals or more.

Calories (kcals) (per 100 gms)

Cereals		Biscuits (sweet)	450
Arrowroot	355	Bread (brown)	244
Barley	361	Bread (white)	245
Biscuits (salt)	336	Cornflakes	368

Custard Powder	354
Macaroni (boiled)	117
Oatmeal	401
Ragi	328
Rice (raw)	345
Rice flakes	346
Rice (puffed)	325
Wheat (whole)	346
Wheat flour	348
Wheat daliya	348

Pulses and Legumes

Bengal gram	372
Bengal gram (roasted)	369
Black gram	347
Green gram	348
Horse gram	321
Red gram (tuvar)	335
Peas (dry)	315
Peas (frozen)	53
Kidney beans (rajma)	346
Soyabean	432
Soya flour	352

Vegetables

Bamboo shoots	43
Beet green	46
Bottlegourd	12
Broad beans	48
Broccoli	23
Brussels sprouts	52
Cabbage	27
Coriander leaves	44
Curry leaves	108
Drumstick leaves	92
Fenugreek leaves (methi)	49
Lettuce	21
Mint	48
Spinach	26
Cluster beans	60
French beans	26
Bittergourd	25
Brinjal	24
Cauliflower	30
Celery	18
Cucumber	13
Drumstick	26
Capsicums	24
Knol-kol	21
Lady'sfinger	35
Leeks	77
Lotus stem	234
Mushrooms	13
Papaya (green)	27
Peas	93
Plantain (flower)	34
Plantain (green)	64
Plantain (stem)	42
Pumpkin (red)	25
Pumpkin (white)	10
Ridgegourd	17
Snakegourd	18
Tinda	21
Tomato (green)	23
Vegetable marrow (lauki)	17
Beetroot	43

Carrot	48
Colocasia	97
Onion (big)	50
Onion (small)	59
Potato	97
Potato (boiled)	80
Potato (roast)	157
Radish	17
Sweet potato	120
Turnip	29
Yam	59

Nuts and Oilseeds

Almond	655
Cashewnut	596
Coconut (dry)	662
Coconut (fresh)	444
Gingelly seeds	563
Groundnut	567
Pistachio	626
Walnut	687

Condiments and Spices

Asafoetida	297
Cardamom	229
Chillies (dry)	246
Chillies (green)	29
Cloves	286
Coriander seeds	288
Cuminseeds	356
Fenugreek seeds	333
Garlic	145
Ginger	67
Mace	437
Mango powder	337
Nutmeg	472
Omum	363
Pepper (dry)	304
Pepper (green)	98
Poppy seeds	408
Tamarind pulp	283
Turmeric	349

Fruits

Apple	59
Apricot	53
Avocado	215
Banana	116
Blackberry	56
Breadfruit	56
Cherries	64
Chikoo	98
Currants	316
Custard apple (sitaphal)	104
Dates (dried)	317
Dates (fresh)	144
Figs	37
Gooseberries	17
Grapes (purple)	58
Grapes (green)	71
Guava	51
Jackfruit	88
Lemon	57
Lime (sweet)	43
Lichi	61
Mango	74
Melon (musk)	17

Melon (water)	16
Olive	103
Orange	48
Papaya	32
Passion fruit	54
Peaches	50
Pears	52
Pineapple	46
Plum	52
Pomegranate	65
Prunes	56
Raisins	308
Raspberries	56
Strawberries	44
Sultanas (dried)	250
Tomato	20
Woodapple	134

Seafood

Bhetki fish	79
Bombay duck	293
Catfish	86
Cod	76
Crab	59
Eel	168
Haddock	73
Halibut	92
Herring	119
Hilsa	273
Lobster (boiled)	119
Mackerel	223
Mussel	81
Pomfret	87
Prawn	89
Rohu	97
Salmon	182
Sardine	101
Shark	93
Shrimp (boiled)	117
Sole	94
Trout	135
Tuna	185

Meat and Poultry

Bacon (lean)	147
Bacon (fat)	747
Brain	110
Duck	130
Egg (duck)	181
Egg (hen)	173
Egg white	36
Egg yolk	339
Fowl	109
Goat meat	118
Ham	120
Heart (lamb)	119
Heart (pig)	93
Kidney (lamb)	90
Lamb (lean)	162
Lamb (fat)	671
Liver (chicken)	135
Liver (goat)	107
Liver (sheep)	150
Pork (lean)	147
Pork (fat)	670
Rabbit	124

Sausage frankfurters	274
Salami	491
Turkey	107
Venison	97

Milk and Its Products

Milk (buffalo)	117
Milk (cow)	67
Milk (goat)	72
Milk (skimmed)	29
Butter	729
Buttermilk	15
Cheese (buffalo milk)	292
Cheese (cow milk)	265
Cheese (cheddar)	406
Cheese (cottage)	96
Cheese spread	283
Curds (cow milk)	60
Ghee	900
Khoya	421
Skimmed milk powder	357
Whole milk powder	496
Yogurt (low fat)	52

Edible Oils and Fats

Cooking oil	900
Hydrogenated oil	900
Lard	891
Margarine	730
Butter	700
Coconut oil	900
Groundnut oil (1tsp)	126
Palm oil	900
Sesame oil	880
Sunflower oil	900

Sugars, Preserves & Desserts

Sugar	398
Glucose (liquid)	318
Honey	319
Jaggery	383
Marmalade	443
Syrup (sugar)	298
Chocolate (milk)	529
Chocolate (plain)	525
Peppermints	392
Bread pudding	297
Fruit salad	80
Gulab jamun	387
Jalebi	494
Jam	260
Jelly	280
Rice kheer	250

Alcoholic Drinks

Beer (100 ml)	25
Brandy (30 ml)	65
Gin (30 ml)	65
Rum (30 ml)	65
Sherry (30 ml)	43
Vodka (30 ml)	65
Whisky (30 ml)	65
Wine (red-100 ml)	68
Wine (white-100 ml)	76

Non-alcoholic Beverages

Apple juice (a glass)	76
Coca-cola (100 ml)	40
Cocoa in milk (1 cup)	224

Coffee (2 tsp sugar)	110
Grape juice (1 glass)	92
Lime juice (1 glass)	47
Milk shake (1 glass)	200
Orange juice (1 glass)	72
Pineapple juice (1 glass)	82
Tea (2 tsp sugar, 1 cup)	110
Tomato juice (1 glass)	28

Miscellaneous

Coconut water	24
Pappad	288
Sago	351
Salt	0
Vinegar	4
Chaat	474
Ketchup	110
Vegetable cutlet (1)	126
Boiled egg (1)	80
Fried egg (1)	107
Omelette	191
Scrambled egg	247
Egg fried rice	208
Pakoras (6)	197
Pasta	86
Samosa (1)	472
Sponge cake	459
Upama	153
Halwa (wheat)	263
Puri (1)	68
Bhelpuri	182
Chapati (2)	202
Dal (1 cup)	80
Idli (rice –2)	130
Idli (semolina – 2)	16
Noodles	390
Ice-cream	185
Biscuits (home made)	463
Paratha (1)	328
Dahi vada (1)	83
Dosa (1)	210
Kachori (1)	190
Naan (1)	336
Cream (fresh)	583
Cream (canned)	237

Diabetics need more nourishing and better balanced diet than normal people due to certain limitations in their metabolism. In trying to normalise blood sugar, essential nutrients required for normal growth should not be compromised.

Special adjustments are required for insulin-dependent patients, eating out, social get-togethers, festivals, illnesses, nausea, diarrhoea, etc.

Generally, a diabetic requires 25-30 kcals per kg, body weight, 1-1.5 gm proteins per kg body weight, 30-50 gm fat, 200-300 gm carbohydrates (starch, not sugar), fibres from fruits, vegetable and cereals, and vitamins and minerals.

Too many calories in your diet worsen your control of diabetes. To reduce the risk of developing coronary heart disease and arterial disease, the amount of fat in the diet should be low. If you need to lose weight, have a carbohydrate diet, which has some bread or potatoes or pasta, or rice or breakfast cereal at each meal, for this has bulk and fibre.

Low calorie 'diet' foods and drinks can be included in your diet to lose weight. These days, doctors do allow a little sugar, to be taken at the end of a high-fibre meal.

Porridge at breakfast is an excellent breakfast cereal for diet control. A sandwich lunch made of whole meal bread can be very healthy. Diet yoghurts make excellent desserts. Low sugar jelly too is a good dessert.

SWEETENING AGENTS

It is very difficult to avoid sweets, especially if you have a 'sweet tooth'. Sugar is the most commonly used sweetening agent. One gram of sugar provides 4 kcals.

Sweetening agents are non-calorific or intense sweetness, or they are calorific sweetness or bulk sweeteners.

Non-calorific Sweeteners

Saccharin: This is an intensely sweet, white, crystalline compound from coal tar and petroleum. People on a low-carbohydrate diet use it as a substitute for sugar, either because they have diabetes or wish to control their intake of calories. It is 350 times sweeter than sugar. It leaves a bitter after taste and is decomposed by heat. It is used in canned fruits and preserves, soft drinks, chewing gums, toothpastes and drugs. Saccharin is added to tea, coffee or a dish after the food or drink is prepared, and not while cooking or boiling.

Aspartame: This is a low-calorie sweetening agent. It is a mixture of amino-acids, and is 180-200 times sweeter than sugar. Unlike saccharin, it does not leave a bitter after taste. In India, it is marketed as Sugar Free and Equal. It does not have a very long shelf life, for after six months, it loses its sweetness.

Calorific Sweeteners

Fructose: This is a type of sugar found naturally in fruit and honey. As this does not need insulin for its metabolism, it is often used as a sweetening agent in diabetic foods.

Sorbitol: This is a chemical related to sugar and alcohol. It is used as a sweetener, substituting for ordinary sugar. It has no significant effect upon the blood glucose level, but has the same calories (4 kcals per kg) as sugar. Anyone wishing to lose weight should not go in for sorbitol. It is poorly absorbed and may have a laxative effect.

Those who wish to eat a fruit can do so, but occasionally, or under a doctor's guidance. Pure, unsweetened fruit juice raises your blood glucose levels. If you eat it as a whole fruit, then it takes time to digest and the effect on blood glucose is quite slow, as it has fibre.

7
FOOD EXCHANGES

Exchanges are portions of carbohydrate foods in the diabetes diet which can be exchanged for one another, that is, one exchange = 10 gm carbohydrate.

You can make your diet interesting if you can grasp the concept of food exchanges. Since the calorie value and the carbohydrate content of cereals are generally the same, these can be interchanged weight for weight. Pulses and legumes have more or less the same composition, hence interchange is allowed. Oil, ghee and vanaspati have also the same fat content, and are interchangeable.

A small banana, a medium-sized apple, an orange, a sweet lime provide 10 gm carbohydrates and can be exchanged.

An exchange is possible within the same group of foodstuffs, e.g., meat can be exchanged with fish, but not fruit. A diabetic can eat biscuits instead of bread for breakfast, but he cannot skip the bread at breakfast and eat an extra chapati at lunch.

No one-exchange group can supply all the nutrients needed for a well-balanced diet. It takes all six of them working together as a team to supply your nutritional needs for good health. The exchanges are:

1. *Milk Exchanges:* Different types of milk and yoghurt.
2. *Vegetable Exchanges:* Some raw vegetables may be used freely, like lettuce, radish, parsley, and cucumber. Starchy vegetables are included in the bread exchange.
3. *Fruit Exchanges:* Fruits that are high in vitamins A and C, and potassium.
4. *Bread Exchanges:* Bread, cereal, and starchy vegetables like potatoes, corn, peas, etc.
5. *Meat Exchanges:* These fall into three groups: lean meat, medium-fat meat, and high-fat meat. The list includes meats, fish, poultry, and other protein-rich foods like cheese, beans and peas.
6. *Fat Exchanges:* Both animal and vegetable fats.

The foods that should be used in a limited way are sugar, candy, soft drinks and some beverages.

Some foods can be used in an unlimited way. These are calorie-free soft drinks, decaffeinated coffee, tea (not too much), boiled meat without fat, seasoning such as lemon, lime, garlic, paprika, cinnamon, vinegar, mint and herbs.

FOOD EXCHANGE LIST

Carbohydrates	**10 gms**	**gm**
Cereals		
Biscuits (sweet)	2	15
Bread	1 small slice	20
Chapati	1 thin, small	15
Cornflakes	4 tbsps	15
Custard powder	3 tbsps	10
Porridge oats (dry)	3 tbsps	15
Rice (cooked)	½ cup	15
Rice flakes (thick)	¼ cup	15
Rice flakes (thin)	½ cup	15

Semolina	1 ½ tbsps	15
Wheat flour	2 ¼ tbsps	15
Wheat (puffed)	4 tbsps	15

Pulses and Legumes

Pulses and legumes	1 ½ tbsps	18

Vegetables

Onion	1 ½ cups, cut	100
Potato (medium-sized pieces)	½ cup	50
Yam	6 pieces, small	60

Fruits

Apple	1 small	80
Apple juice	1/3 cup	87
Banana	1 small	40
Chikoo	1 small	50
Dates (dried)	2	15
Grapes	12	75
Guava (small pieces)	1 cup	100
Mango (small pieces)	½ cup	60
Orange	1 medium	75
Pear	1 small	70
Peach	1 medium	120
Pineapple	1 slice, ½" thick	100
Pineapple juice	1/3 cup	90
Strawberries	15 large	180
Sweet lime	1 medium	100
Watermelon (small chunks)	2 cups	300

Beverages

Bournvita	2 tsps	15
Cocoa	5 tsps	30
Horlicks	2 tsps	15

Miscellaneous		
Sago	1 tbsp	12
Sugar	1 tsp	10
Protein		
Cheese (grated)	2 ½ tbsps	18
Coconut (tender)	1 ¼ tbsps, grated	
Ghee	1 tsp	5
Groundnut (powdered)	1 ½ tbsps	13
Mayonnaise	1 tsp	5
Oil	1 tsp	5
Vanaspati	1 tsp	5

Cereals and pulses can be exchanged weight for weight.

STANDARD INDIAN DIET (1500 kcal) (in gms)

Breakfast	**kcal**	**Carbohydrate**	**Protein**	**Fat**
Porridge (20 gm)	68	13.8	2.4	0.3
or 1 slice bread (30 gm)	70	15.0	2.4	0.3
Egg (1)	78	-	6.0	6.0
or paneer (30 gm)	79	0.3	5.5	6.2
or cheese (25 gm)	87	1.6	6.0	6.2
Bread slice (1)	70	15.0	2.4	0.3
or chapatti (20 gm)	68	13.8	2.4	0.3
or idli (1)	69	13.0	2.9	0.2
Milk (1cup)	114	7.7	5.5	7.0
Mid-morning				
Tea/coffee				
Fruits/biscuits	70	12.0	1.0	3.0
Lunch				
Salad (25 gm)	35	6.0	3.0	—
Mixed vegetables (100 gms)	35	7.0	2.0	—
Dal (30 gm)	100	17.0	6.7	0.6
or paneer (35 gm)	93	0.4	6.4	7.3
or mutton (50 gm)	97	—	9.3	6.7
Chicken (70 gm)	105	—	17.0	4.0

or fish (100 gm)	91	—	20.0	—
Chapati (2)	136	27.6	4.8	0.6
Curd (130 ml)	80	5.3	3.8	4.8
Tea				
Fruits/biscuits	70	16.0	1.0	—
or glucose	68	10.8	1.0	2.2
or salted	80	8.2	1.0	4.4
Dinner				
Soup	10	2.5	—	—
Salad (125 gm)	35	6.0	3.0	—
Vegetable mixed (100 gms)	35	7.0	2.0	—
Dal (30 gm)	100	17.0	6.7	0.6
Curd	80	5.3	3.8	4.8
Chapati	136	27.6	4.8	0.6
Milk (bed time)	114	7.7	5.5	7.0

Note:

1) This diet contains 215 gms carbohydrates, 70 gms protein, 40 gms fat, 500 ml milk and 15 gm oil.

PROTEIN EXCHANGE EQUIVALENT OF ONE EGG (6.4 gms protein)

Food	Quantity (gms)	Kcal	Proteins (gms)
Egg (large)	45	78	6.4
Cow's milk	200 ml	135	6.4
Buffalo's milk	150 ml	175	6.4
Homogenised milk	150 ml	100	6.4
Skimmed milk	250 ml	72	6.4
Paneer (cow's milk)	35	93	6.4
Paneer (buffalo's milk)	50	146	6.7
Cheese	25	87	6.0
Chicken (fryer)	25	27	6.4
Chicken (broiler)	25	38	6.4
Liver (goat)	30	32	6.0

Kidney	40	42	6.8
Brain	65	81	6.5
Mutton	35	78	6.5
Pork (lean muscle)	30	34	5.6
Sausages	60	270	6.6
Bacon (fried)	25	151	6.2
Ham	25	100	6.0
Fish (skinless, boneless)	35	31	6.4
Crab muscles (cooked 40 gm)	70	41	6.2
Prawns	35	31	6.7
Soyabean	15	65	6.4
Average dal	30	104	6.4
Peanut butter	30	93	6.4
Chana (roasted)	30	110	6.4
Rajma	30	104	6.8
Green peas (fresh)	90	84	6.5

Note: Food in italics have higher fat content, hence to be avoided or adjusted.

CARBOHYDRATE EXCHANGE EQUIVALENT OF ONE CHAPATI (20 gm flour)

Food	Quantity (gms)	Kcal	Carbohydrates (gms)
Cereals			
Flour (thin, small chapati)	20	68	13.9
Raw rice milled (1 cup)	20	68	15.6
Bread, white (1 large slice)	28.5	70	14.8
Bread, brown (1 slice)	28.5	70	13.9
Biscuits, salted (4)	12	65	6.6
Biscuits, sweet (2)	15	68	10.8
Oats porridge (2/3 cup)	20	68	12.6
Maize (1 ½ roti) or cornflakes 2/3 cup	20	68	13.2
Popcorn (1 ½ cups)	15	67	9.0

Rice flakes	20	68	15.5
Rice (puffed)	20	65	14.7
Wheat dalia	20	68	14.0
Sponge cake, plain (1 ¼" of 8" cake)	25	73	13.5
Wheat suji	20	68	14.2
Dal and Beans			
Dal	20	68	11.6
Rajma	20	68	12.1
Kabuli chana or Bengal gram	20	68	12.2
Baked beans (in tomato sauce ½ cup)	60	73	13.8
Vegetables			
Carrots	140	70	14.8
Colocasia/potato	70	70	15.4
Salads	250	70	10.0
Leafy vegetable	150	66	10.5
Beetroot	160	70	14.1
Lotus root	130	70	14.7
Onion	150	75	16.6
Radish (2 large)	400	60	13.6
Sweet potato	60	68	16.9
Yam	85	68	15.6
Fruits			
Apple (1 medium)	120	72	16.0
Banana (1 small)	60	65	16.3
Peach (2 small)	150	75	15.7
Pear (2 small)	125	65	14.9
Plum (2 medium)	125	65	13.9
Papaya (1/4 medium)	225	72	16.2
Orange (2 medium)	150	72	16.4
Musambi	150	63	14.0
Malta orange	200	72	15.6

Green grapes (1 small bunch)	100	71	16.5
Watermelon (3" slice)	450	72	14.8
Musk melon (1/2" medium)	400	68	14.0
Lichi (5-6)	125	73	17.0
Guava (1 medium)	125	64	14.0

Note: Items in italics have high carbohydrate content.

FAT EXCHANGE (15 gm fat) (1 tbsp ghee)

Food	Quantity (gms)	Kcal	Proteins (gms)
Butter	20	140	15.0
Cream	40	135	15.8
Mayonnaise	20	138	15.0
Ghee	15	135	15.0
Vanaspati	15	135	15.0
Cooking oil	15	135	15.0

FIBRE CONTENT OF FOODS (100 gms)

Food	Fibre gms.
Pulses & Legumes	
Green gram (moong, whole)	4.1
Green gram split	0.8
Black gram (urad dal)	0.9
Bengal gram (chana dal)	1.2
Lentil (masur dal)	0.7
Red gram (tuvar dal)	1.5
Soyabeans	3.1
Vegetables	
Cabbage	1.0
Cauliflower	1.2
Carrots	1.2

Coriander leaves	1.2
Cucumber	0.4
Brinjals	1.3
Bittergourd	0.8
Drumsticks	5.0
Lady'sfingers	1.2
Leeks	1.3
Lettuce	0.5
Mint	2.0
Fenugreek leaves	1.1
French beans	1.8
Beetroot	1.0
Onions (baby)	0.6
Onions	0.6
Green peas	4.0
Potatoes	0.4
Sweet potatoes	0.8
Radish	0.8
Spinach	0.6
Tomato	0.8
Tomato juice	0.25

Fruits

Apples	1.0
Apricots	1.0
Bananas	0.4
Cherries	0.4
Currants	1.0
Dates (fresh)	4.0
Figs	2.2
Green grapes	3.0
Guava	5.2
Jackfruit	1.0
Lemon	2.0
Lichi	0.8

Mango	0.7
Melon (water)	0.2
Orange	0.3
Papaya	0.8
Peaches	1.2
Pears	1.0
Pineapple	0.5
Plums	0.4
Pomegranate	5.1
Raisins	1.1
Custard apple	3.1
Chikoo	2.6
Strawberries	1.1
Cereals	
Barley	4.0
Oatmeal	3.5
Raw rice (milled)	0.2
Raw rice (unmilled)	0.6
Wheat flour	2.0
Maida	0.3
Bread (wheat)	0.2
Wheat gram	1.4
Nuts and Seeds	
Almonds	2.0
Cashewnuts	1.0
Coconut (dry)	7.0
Groundnuts (roasted)	3.0
Pistachio	2.0
Walnuts	3.0

STANDARD DIABETIC DIET (1500 kcal) (in gms)

Food	Qty.	Kcal	Protein	Fat	Carbo.
Cow's milk	500	335	16.0	20.5	22.0
Egg (1)	45	78	6.0	6.0	—
Dal	60	200	13.5	1.2	35.0
Bread	60	140	4.8	0.6	30.0
Biscuits (salt)	15	68	1.0	4.5	7.5
Wheat flour	80	272	8.0	2.0	56.0
Leafy vegetable	150	66	5.0	1.0	9.0
Salad	250	70	8.0	—	27.0
Vegetables	200	70	—	—	—
Fruits	100-150	70	—	—	15.7
Oil	15	135	—	15.0	—
Total		1504	62.3	50.8	202.2

What you should remember is that sugar in any form— sweet, ice-creams, kulfi, chocolates, etc.—should be avoided. Instead, take desserts that are low in calorie and have artificial sweeteners.

Avoid vegetables that are rich in high starch content, like potatoes, colocasia, sweet, sweet potatoes, yam, etc. Instead, consume green vegetables rich in fibre, like leeks, bittergourd and bottlegourd, lettuce, beans, brinjals, lady'sfingers, cabbage, cauliflower, carrot, soyabeans, drumsticks. You can also take the following vegetables in moderate quantity: peas, beetroot, jackfruit, and onions.

Instead of refined cereals like semolina, maida, refined wheat floor and rice, you can substitute wheat flour with bran, and rice after eliminating its starch water.

Skimmed milk and its products are better than whole milk and its products. Oil can be substituted for ghee and butter. Dry chapatis are preferable to parathas, puris, samosas, pakoras, etc.

Substitute high sugary or starchy fruits like banana, chikoo, grapes, lichi, mango, etc., with orange, watermelon, sweet lime, apple, papaya, etc.

It is better to consume egg white, meat like fish, chicken, lamb rather than ham, egg yolk, sausages, organ meat like liver, kidney, brain, etc.

If you do need to take alcohol, restrict it to whisky and brandy in moderation rather than consume beer or wines.

Weighing Food

A diabetic need not have food specially cooked for him. He can pick up a suitable portion from what has been cooked for the rest of the family.

Those foodstuffs, which have low carbohydrate and low calories are known as free foods. These can be consumed without weighing, and without restrictions.

Weighing foods from time to time is a good practice. A cup of raw rice or flour can be weighed, and then you can assess how much rice can be cooked, or how many chapatis can be made. In this way, you know how much flour or raw rice is required for a diabetic.

COMMONLY USED FOODSTUFFS (HOUSEHOLD MEASURES)

Foods	Measure	Weight	Kcal
Cereals			
Bread	1 slice small	20	50
Bread	1 slice large	30	75
Cornflour	4 ½ tbsps	30	100
Macaroni (cut)	1 cup	50	175
Noodles	1 cup	50	175
Semolina	3 tbsps	30	100
Rice flakes (thick)	½ cup	30	100

Rice flakes (thin)	1 cup	30	100
Rice (puffed)	1 cup	10	33
Wheat flour (with bran)	4 ½ tbsps	30	100
Wheat flour (refined)	4 tbsps	30	100
Rice	¼ cup	30	100
Pulses & Legumes			
Pulses/legumes	¼ cup	30	100
Bengal gram (roasted)	¼ cup	16	60
Vegetables			
Leafy vegetables (chopped)	1 cup	25	10
Other vegetables (chopped)	1 cup	50	10
Onion (chopped)	1 ½ cups	100	50
Potato (medium-sized pieces)	½ cup	50	45
Fruits			
Apple	1 small	80	54
Apple juice	1/3 cup	87	58
Banana	1 small	60	65
Chickoo	1 small	50	98
Dates (dried)	2	50	108
Grapes	12	75	55
Guava (small pieces)	1 cup	100	50
Mango (small pieces)	½ cup	60	
Orange	1 medium	45	36
Pear	1 small	70	32
Peach	1 medium	120	65
Pineapple	1 slice, ½"thick	100	46
Strawberries	15 large	180	75
Sweet lime	1 medium	100	36

Water melon (small chunks)	2 cups	300	60
Dry Fruits			
Dates	5, without seeds	30	45
Raisins	1 tbsp	10	30
Nuts and Oilseeds			
Almond	8 medium	10	65
Cashewnut	5	10	55
Coconut, dry (grated)	1 tbsp	10	45
Coconut, dry (grated)	1 tbsp	9	50
Walnut	2 without shell	10	70
Non-vegetarian			
Bacon	1 slice (raw)	7	48
Chicken	1 leg	105	55
Mutton	1 piece (lemon size)	20	25
Pomfret	1 large piece	50	45
Egg (hen)	1 whole	55	65
Milk & its Products			
Milk, buffalo	1 cup	150 ml	140
Butter	1 tsp	5	40
Ghee	1 tsp	5	45
Oils			
Hydrogenated fat	1 tsp	5	45
Vegetable oil	1 tsp	5	45
Miscellaneous			
Jaggery	1 tsp	7.5	29
Sago	2 tbsps	25	85
Sugar	1 tbsp	15	60

Eating Out

Sometimes, it becomes very difficult to decide what to eat when eating out with friends who have made a special effort to prepare delicious food, especially if the spread turns out to be unsuitable for a diabetic. Should he refuse a delectable pudding and offend his hostess, or should he have a large helping and forget for once all about his diabetes? It will be less embarrassing for him to warn his friend about his conditions in advance, than to be faced with a dilemma later on. Restaurants or takeaways should not be so much of a problem as one has a wide choice of dishes to choose from.

As a diabetic normally knows what foods should be avoided, he would be able to judge his portions visually. As a rule, it would be wise of him to avoid foodstuffs of unknown composition. If he has to eat out very often, he should stick to what is familiar to him rather than go in for something, which sounds novel and appetising, but may have all the wrong ingredients in it.

Thin soup, clear broth, unsweetened tomato juice, radish, carrot, green salad, tomato, cucumber are safe to eat, while creamy soups and fried hors d'ouvres should be avoided. You can also have chapati, plain rice, cooked meat, cooked pulses and legumes, cooked vegetables having less than 10 per cent carbohydrates. Avoid eating parathas, fried rice, fried meat, fried chicken, etc. Plain fruit is better than sweets, canned fruits with sugar, desserts of unknown composition.

Adaptation of Conventional Recipes

You can change a conventional recipe to suit your needs. You can use a sweetener where sugar can be dispensed with; you can substitute a high calorie food for one that is suitable for you, i.e., low in calories; you can use cauliflowers instead of potato, or use herbs of garnishing instead of mayonnaise or salad oil. You can bake, grill or steam instead of frying.

You can use pepper, chillies, spices, mustard, curry powder, parsley, turmeric, yeast, cardamom, garlic, coriander, ginger, gelatin, vanilla, lemon and orange peels, lemon juice, clear stock, cloves, citric acid, tomato, radish, mushrooms, etc., for garnishing or to add to your dishes.

8

MAKING HEALTHY FOOD CHOICES

Knowing what to eat can be confusing. Everywhere you turn, there is news about what is or isn't good for you. Some basic principles have weathered the fad diets, and have stood the test of time. Here are a few tips on making healthful food choices for you and your entire family.

- Eat lots of vegetables and fruits. Try picking from the rainbow of colors available to maximize variety. Eat non-starchy vegetables such as spinach, carrots, broccoli or green beans with meals.
- Choose whole grain foods over processed grain products. Try brown rice with your stir fry or whole wheat spaghetti with your favorite pasta sauce.
- Include dried beans (like kidney or pinto beans) and lentils into your meals.
- Include fish in your meals 2-3 times a week.
- Choose lean meats like cuts of beef and pork that end in "loin" such as pork loin and sirloin. Remove the skin from chicken and turkey.
- Choose non-fat dairy such as skim milk, non-fat yogurt and non-fat cheese.

- Choose water and calorie-free "diet" drinks instead of regular soda, fruit punch, sweet tea and other sugar-sweetened drinks.
- Choose liquid oils for cooking instead of solid fats that can be high in saturated and trans fats. Remember that fats are high in calories. If you're trying to lose weight, watch your portion sizes of added fats.
- Cut back on high calorie snack foods and desserts like chips, cookies, cakes, and full-fat ice cream.
- Eating too much of even healthful foods can lead to weight gain. Watch your portion sizes.

Want more information on foods that are healthier, or how to establish a plan for eating healthy foods? Let the American Diabetes Association help point you in the right direction.

9

SWEETENERS AND DESSERTS

If you have diabetes, that doesn't mean you can't eat sweets. People with diabetes can eat desserts, use sweeteners, and still keep their blood glucose (sugar) levels in their target range. These options are available for sweetening your foods:

- Sugar and other sweeteners with calories including honey, brown sugar, molasses, fructose, cane sugar, and confectioners sugar
- Reduced-calorie sweeteners including erythritol, hydrogenated starch hydrolysates, isomalt, lactitol, maltitol, mannitol, sorbitol, and xylitol
- Low-calorie sweeteners such as ascelfume potassium, aspartame, saccharin and sucralose.

Sugar and Other Sweeteners with Calories

In the past, people with diabetes were warned to completely avoid sugar. Experts thought that eating sugar would rapidly increase blood glucose, resulting in levels that were too high. Some people even thought that eating sugar caused diabetes, an idea that we now know isn't true.

Research has shown that the total amount of carbohydrate affects blood glucose levels the most. But, the type of carbohydrate (e.g. sugar vs. starch) can also affect blood glucose levels. Now experts agree you can eat foods with sugar as long as you work them into your meal plan as you would any other carb-containing food. The same guidelines apply to other sweeteners with calories, including brown sugar, honey, and molasses.

Of course, most sweets and desserts don't provide the important vitamins and minerals found in more healthful foods, so you'll want to make sure you're still getting the nutrients you need. Many sweets, in addition to having carbs, are also high in fat and calories.

10

SPECIMEN DIET FOR DIABETICS

1. Vegetarian (1,200 kcals)

Breakfast

Milk	¾ cup	112 ml
Tea/coffee (no sugar)	1 cup	37 ml
(with milk)	¼ cup	
Bread	4 small slices	80 gm

Mid-morning Snack

Orange	1	

Lunch

Rice (uncooked)	¼ cup	30 gm
Wheat flour	4 ½ tbsps	30 gms
Vegetables (less than 10% carbo.)	unlimited	
Buttermilk	unlimited	
Oil for cooking	4 ½ tsps	22 gms

Tea Time

Tea/coffee (sugarless) with milk	¼ cup	37 ml
Marie biscuits	3	

Supper

Same as lunch		
Curds	¼ cup	37 ml

Bed Time

Milk	1 cup	150 ml
Marie biscuits	1	

2. Non-vegetarian (1,200 kcal)

Breakfast

Milk	¾ cup	112 ml
Tea/coffee (sugarless, milk 1/4cup)	1 cup	37 ml
Bread	3 small slices	60 gm
Egg white	1	

Mid-morning Snack

Orange	1	

Lunch

Rice (uncooked)	¼ cup	30 gms
Wheat flour	6 tbsps	40 gm
Mutton (boneless)	2 pieces (lemon-sized)	40 gm
Vegetables (less than 10% carbo.)	unlimited	
Buttermilk	unlimited	
Oil for cooking	4 ½ tsps	22 gm

Tea Time

Tea/coffee (sugarless, with milk 1/4 cup)	1 cup	37 ml
Marie biscuits	3	

Supper

Rice (uncooked)	¼ cup	30 gm
Wheat flour	4 ½ tbsps	30 gms
Pulse/legumes	¼ cup	30 gms
Vegetables (less than 10% carbo.)	unlimited	
Curds	¼ cup	37 ml
Buttermilk	unlimited	

Bed Time

Milk	1 cup	150 ml
Marie biscuits	1	22 gm

3. Vegetarian (1,700 kcal)

Breakfast

Milk	¾ cup	112 ml
Tea/coffee (sugarless, with milk 1/4 cup) 1 cup	37 ml	
Bread	4 thin slices	80 gm

Mid-morning Snack

Orange	1	

Lunch

Rice (uncooked)	¼ cup	30 gms
Wheat flour	9 tbsps	60 gm
Pulses/legumes	1/3 cup	40 gm
Vegetables (less than 10% carbo.)	unlimited	
Buttermilk	unlimited	
Oil for cooking	6 tsps	30 gm

Tea Time

Tea/coffee (sugarless, with milk 1/4 cup)	1 cup	37 ml
Marie biscuits	3	

Supper

Same as lunch		
Curds	¼ cup	37 ml

Bed Time

Milk	1 cup	150 ml
Marie biscuits	1	

Non-vegetarian (1,700 kcal)

Breakfast		
Milk	¾ cup	112 ml
Tea/coffee (sugarless, with milk 1/4 cup)	1 cup	37 ml
Bread	4 small slices	80 gm
Egg white	1	
Mid-morning Snack		
Orange	1	
Lunch		
Rice (uncooked)	3¼ cups	30 gms
Wheat flour	11 tbsps	80 gm
Mutton (boneless)	3 pieces (lemon-sized)	60 gm
Vegetables (less than 10% carbo.)	unlimited	
Buttermilk	unlimited	
Oil for cooking	6 tsps	
Tea Time		
Tea/coffee (sugarless, with milk 1/4 cup)	1 cup	37 ml
Marie biscuits	3	
Supper		
Rice (uncooked)	¼ cup	30 gm
Wheat flour	9 tbsps	60 gms
Pulse / legumes	1/3 cup	40 gms
Vegetables (less than 10% carbo.)	unlimited	
Curds	¼ cup	37 ml
Buttermilk	unlimited	
Bed Time		
Milk	1 cup	150 ml
Marie biscuits	1	22 gm

11
EXERCISE PLANNING

Exercise is one of the fundamentals of diabetes control. Modern transport has deprived many people the habit of walking which is one of the best and safest forms of exercise.

Some adults, particularly those who lead sedentary lives, become concerned that their daily routine does not provide them with enough exercise. Such people, especially diabetics, can develop habits to keep them in good condition. Walking, playing golf, climbing stairs, sports, etc., are useful in maintaining fitness.

The kind of recreation or exercise that is best depends on a person's state of health, the type of food he eats and the rest or sleep that he gets. The exercises should be done regularly. A little daily exercise is better than a sporadic burst of activity.

Benefits of Exercise

Total lack of exercise can have a debilitating effect on the body. If the energy supported by food is not all used, the surplus is converted into fat. The muscles may weaken and soften through lack of use, and the circulation may become sluggish.

Exercise helps to develop muscles, maintain muscle tone and improve posture. Breathing is deepened, making it easier for the body to obtain oxygen, and to rid itself of carbon dioxide, and muscular movement quickens the circulation.

Combined with a sensible diet, exercise can help to regulate body weight. It can burn up the extra calories, and help in controlling weight. It makes insulin more effective in lowering your blood glucose level, and helping in the entry of glucose into the cells. It also helps in alleviating hypertension and physical tension, increases the efficiency of your lungs and heart, and reduces the cholesterol level in the bloodstream. Whether healthy or diabetic, regular exercise gives a feeling of well being.

Since diabetics, blood vessel disease and obesity are closely interrelated, exercise has a special significance to a person who has diabetes.

When you exercise, the assimilation of glucose in the body is easier. The exercising muscles react better to insulin than muscles at rest. The overall result of exercise is the lowering of the blood glucose level. However, only if insulin is available are the benefits of exercise enjoyed. Otherwise, the strenuous physical activity actually increases the blood glucose level, and may lead to production of ketosis.

Hazards of Exercise

When the blood glucose level is over 300 mg per cent in insulin-dependent patients and over 40 mg per cent in non-insulin dependent diabetics, exercising can become hazardous, as the blood glucose level will rise further.

In a normal person, during exercise, the liver releases stored glucose. The muscles use this glucose as fuel, when the insulin circulating is adequate. A high blood glucose before exercise means that the circulating insulin in the blood cannot match the blood glucose level. In such situations, the blood glucose level increases further with the glucose released from the liver.

When ketosis is present, avoid exercises, for it worsens, the blood glucose level gets aggravated, and diabetic ketoacidosis gets precipitated. If you have vigorous walking, running or jogging. If your feet are numb, swimming is good. Avoid walking with an open wound, a painful corn or a callus of the foot.

While exercising, if you experience discomfort in the chest, jaws or arms, severe breathlessness, dizziness, marked fatigue, or irregularity of heartbeat, report to your doctor at once. If you have high blood pressure, do not undertake any vigorous type of exercises.

If you have been laser treated for retinal disease, avoid lifting weights. Do not consume alcohol immediately after exercise.

Extreme climates can be hazardous for exercises. In hot, humid weather, there are chances of your developing hypoglycaemia or dehydration, while in winter frostbite and cracked skin can result. At such times, exercise indoors is advisable.

Exercise Programme

There are many different systems of exercise, but they all have the same general purpose: to loosen up the body and then exercise each part in turn.

It may be advisable for young diabetics to begin exercising under the supervision of a trained instructor. It is important to begin by exercising gently and then working up to a level of activity that does not put an undue strain on the body. Always stop exercising when you feel tired, to avoid exhausting yourself.

Any kind of exercise requires a certain amount of self-discipline. Many people who would like to be fit begin exercising, but after an initial enthusiasm, lose interest in their programme. Before starting, you should realise that exercises are repetitious and, therefore, are almost bound to the tedious. Moreover, they are effective only if you are prepared to do them daily for an indefinite period.

Exercise is not a guarantee of longevity, nor does it prevent the ailments of old age. Embarking on a course of strenuous exercise in, say, the forties or fifties, after a period of inactivity, may have the opposite effect. It may drain away reserves of energy and put an intolerable strain on the body. So one should check with one's doctor before setting out with any form of exercise.

A young diabetic can run, bicycle and play tennis, badminton and other games. A middle-aged or elderly diabetic should exercise moderately and only when judged fit by the doctor. Walking, by far, is the best exercise for them.

Young women can take part in games and physical exercises, which will not affect their menstruation. Pregnant women should be careful with their exercises, and not indulge in competitive sports.

(12)

EXERCISE FOR INSULIN-DEPENDENT DIABETICS

You can avoid hypoglycaemia and hyperglycaemia, if you are an insulin dependent diabetic, by understanding how exercise helps or worsens your health. Either of the setbacks can result if you do not plan your exercise programme properly. You have to adhere loosely to your daily schedule, by eating your meals, taking your insulin, and exercising at the same each day.

Since working muscles use more energy than relaxed muscles, exercise increases your muscle's demand for glucose. The glucose circulating in the bloodstream produces the energy. This helps in lowering your blood sugar level.

When you take insulin injections and exercise, the site of the injection shows easier absorption of insulin by your body, for example, injection on your thigh shows increased absorption rate of insulin when you run or jog. This is not beneficial as the injected insulin may act too quickly on your system. Therefore, your physician can guide you about the injection sites in your body that have least exercise.

In many cases, it is beneficial to have increased insulin absorption as it may decrease the amount of insulin you have to take. Care is needed to carefully balance the insulin with the food you eat and the amount of exercise you get. For overweight diabetics, the physician may recommend that you lower your insulin injections rather than increase your food intake. This allows you to burn more calories with no extra food, and thus help in weight reduction.

The best time to exercise is between half an hour and two hours after a meal, as the blood sugar is higher than at any other time. If you feel you need some extra food before exercises, eat it 15 minutes before you exercise. When you exercise vigorously, you may require extra food every half hour.

Sometimes you may notice signs of hypoglycaemia soon after exercising, at such a time you may require food. So when you go on long treks or biking or bicycle ride, carry extra food. Blood sugar that has been depleted by too much exercise can be replenished immediately by taking a sugar cube, or a hard candy, or orange juice. If you do become hypoglycaemic, eat extra food till the symptoms subside. After your blood sugar has returned to normal, if it is not near meal time, it is better to eat some complex carbohydrates, such as bread or cereal, to keep your blood glucose level balanced.

Insulin may peak anywhere from about two to 12 hours after injection, depending on the kind you inject. It is not good to exercise at such a time as the combination of exercise and high insulin level could lead to hypoglycaemia.

(13)

EXERCISES FOR NON INSULIN DEPENDENT DIABETICS

For a person who is non-insulin dependent diabetic (NIDD) and is overweight, his main aim would be to lose weight through exercise. The following table shows approximately how many calories you can lose while exercising:

Activity	Calories Burnt Per Hour
Light	***(50-199)***
Sleeping or lying down	80
Sitting	100
Driving a car	120
Standing	140
Housework	180
Moderate	***(200-299)***
Walking (4.25 kms)	210
Cycling (8.25 kms)	210
Gardening	230
Canoeing	230
Golf	250
Lawn mowing	250
Bowling	270

Activity	Calories
Marked	***(300-399)***
Fencing	300
Rowing (4.25 kms)	300
Swimming (400 meters)	300
Walking (6 kms)	300
Badminton	350
Horse riding	350
Volleyball	350
Roller-skating	350
Table tennis	360
Vigorous	***(more than 400)***
Ice-skating (16 km)	400
Woodcutting	400
Tennis	420
Hill climbing (30.5 metres)	480
Skiing (16 km)	490
Squash	600
Handball	600
Cycling (21 km)	660
Running (16 km)	900

Hypertension, Cholesterol and Diabetes

Hypertension is high blood pressure. The normal pumping action of the heart generates in the blood a fluid pressure sufficient to force it round the circulation. In hypertension, this pressure is too high for the body's normal needs.

Hypertension throws a strain on the heart, which has to pump harder to get the blood round the body. It also gradually damages the small blood vessels in the kidneys and the eyes. A cycle of events may develop in which the kidneys, damaged by high blood pressure, cause the pressure to rise even further. This needs urgent attention.

Exercise can also lower your blood pressure, and help in keeping at large any coronary artery disease. Apart from hypertension, other factors that contribute to coronary heart disease are smoking, obesity, high cholesterol level, stress and diabetes. If you have diabetes, you will do your utmost in your capacity to avoid the other contributing factors for coronary artery disease.

High blood pressure should be carefully controlled in diabetes in order to prevent a stroke, a strain on the heart, damage to the kidneys, retina and arteries. Some anti-hypertensive drugs can worsen diabetes, while some can increase the blood flow to the lower limbs, or even cause impotence.

Cholesterol is a substance present in the blood, brain and all other tissues throughout the body, as well as in many foods. The body, chiefly in the liver and adrenal glands, manufactures it. Chemically it is a steroid.

Exercise and diet may help you in lowering the high cholesterol content in your body. This is essential as a high cholesterol level has been associated with atherosclerosis. In atherosclerosis, the lining of the arteries is covered with fatty deposits that contain large amounts of cholesterol. In some cases, a significant rise in the quantity of cholesterol in the blood precedes the appearance of these deposits. The deposits attract compounds of calcium, which also thicken the walls of the arteries, and make them hard and inelastic.

The hardening of the arteries increases the chances of hypertension, which in turn can cause further atherosclerosis. Diabetes can increase the likelihood of both these. Exercise may reduce the blood cholesterol level, for by exercising, the amount of high-density lipoproteins in your bloodstream increases, thus removing cholesterol from your body.

14

SPORTS AND DIABETICS

If you are good in a particular sports, diabetes should not stop you becoming a great sportsperson in your field. People with diabetes have reached the top in many sports.

The extra energy used in competitive sports increases the risk of a hypo. A young diabetic participating in vigorous activities like sports should take extra carbohydrate before a match or any other sports period, like a couple of sandwiches or biscuits. At half time, he will probably need another snack, and he must carry glucose tablets in his pocket.

An active diabetic needs to be careful about what he eats after the game has finished. The effect of exercise on the body can last well after the exercise has stopped as the muscles are restocking their energy stores with glycogen. Very often the blood glucose drops two or more hours after the exercise period. He may then need a snack or if he is due for a meal anyway he may need a slightly larger one than usual. It would also be a good idea for him to have a larger than usual bed-time snack if he has been exercising in the afternoon or evening.

Another way to reduce a hypo diving exercise is to decrease the amount of insulin beforehand. So if a diabetic is playing some sports in the morning, he could reduce his morning dose of quick acting insulin by half.

Though a hypo during athletics and most team games can be inconvenient, a hypo while swimming can be more serious. You have to be sensible about it and should follow certain simple rules with complete safety:

1. Never swim alone.
2. Inform your companions, or teacher, if in school, to pull you out of the water if they see you behaving oddly, or in difficulties.
3. Keep glucose tablets beside the pool.
4. When you feel the first signs of a hypo, do not ignore it, but get out of the water fast.

The vast majority of sports are perfectly safe for people with diabetes. In some sports, like motor racing, the risk of serious injury in the case of a hypo is even greater. Hence, diabetics on insulin are generally discouraged from participating. That does not mean a total ban, depending on whether you are a chronic diabetic case, your age and sex, etc.

When you are jogging or running, keep in mind the following rules:

1. Wear comfortable clothes.
2. Wear proper running shoes, and watch out for blisters.
3. Start with very short runs, and gradually increase the mileage and speed.
4. Aim at training thrice a week.
5. While regular running reduces the average daily insulin dose by about 25 per cent, in training, you will probably need less insulin even on days that you are not running. Once you are out of training then once again more insulin will be needed.

6. During the run you will need to take carbohydrate, and glucose is less likely to cause stomach cramp than a bar of chocolate.
7. Before and after each run, measure blood glucose levels, and keep a careful record of its value, the distance run, the time taken to run it, and the time since the last insulin injection. This will help you in assessing your likely glucose needs for future runs.
8. After the end of a marathon race the blood glucose tends to rise, and you will probably need a small dose of insulin to counteract this.

15

PREGNANCY AND DIABETES

Diabetes spares neither of the sexes, but it poses some special problems. It has a particular affinity for women, but the reasons for this are not known fully. Endocrine and metabolic factors are certainly involved in childbearing and menopause. Mothers more than non-mothers are susceptible to the disease. After the age of 45, women became twice as susceptible as men.

For physiological and other everyday demands made upon the woman, she must take greater care in managing the disease than a man. But the most unique complication of all that adds to the problems of her diabetes is that of pregnancy.

The problems of pregnancy as they affect the diabetes are not particularly complex but they do need careful attention. A woman with diabetes should plan her pregnancy. Raising a family in her early twenties is better than late in life, and she must ensure that her diabetes is well controlled before she becomes pregnant. Glycated haemoglobin test is valuable in this context, as it indicates control of diabetes in the preceding three or four months to pregnancy.

Care during Pregnancy

A diabetic woman will face more stresses and strains during pregnancy than non-diabetic women. She, like other normal women, will also contend with uncertainties, occasional discomfort, morning sickness, and chances of bladder infections, varicose veins and weight gain. She may, at times, feel irritable and depressed for no apparent reason.

For women who become pregnant when their control is poor, there will be an added risk of congenital abnormalities in their babies, some of which may be detectable by ultrasound very early in pregnancy when termination is possible if a major defect is found. Even when there is no defect, the outcome of the pregnancy will still be dictated by the mother's degree of control during her 40 weeks of pregnancy and during labour and delivery.

While all 40 weeks of your pregnancy are important to your baby's growth and development, the first 12 weeks are the most crucial time for normal foetal organ development. So long as control remains perfect, there is no need for hospitalisation. With the excellent control that is now possible, the baby will develop normally, and the pregnancy can be allowed to go its natural 40 weeks term.

Good blood glucose control is the most important goal during pregnancy, and with home blood glucose monitoring this can be achieved in the majority of women. With recent advances in technology, self-testing of blood glucose has become a practical proposition. With this technique, it is possible to achieve a better control of diabetes by adjusting food intake, and through exercise and medication. It facilitates flexibility in your lifestyle.

During the first trimester, you should eat enough food for you and your baby, but avoid high blood sugar and insulin reactions. Your physician will put you on a diet that is higher in calories and particularly in protein, which is essential for healthy development of tissues in your baby. Trying to shed off weight during pregnancy is not recommended, as the baby may then not receive enough nutrients for its healthy growth. Depending on your height and body build, you can expect to put on 10-12 kgs of weight.

The diet should be adequate to avoid ketones in the urine.

There will be more glucose than usual in your urine, even if your blood sugar is not higher than before. This does not indicate that your diabetes is not under control. During pregnancy, what is important is to test for ketones whose presence may indicate difficulties for mother and baby.

It is safer to periodically check your eyes and kidneys to eliminate any complications during pregnancy. Urine cultures are also essential as they can indicate the presence of asymptomatic (no symptoms) urinary tract infection, which are common in all pregnant women.

Those without diabetes generally visit their obstetrician once a month, and later, once a week. A diabetic would need to be examined weekly throughout her pregnancy.

The optimum glucose levels during pregnancy are 70-100 mg per cent in fasting state, and less than 120 mg per cent, two hours after lunch. With ultrasonography, it is possible to assess the growth and size of the foetus at intervals, and to eliminate birth defects, accurately and safely during pregnancy. It is also now possible to monitor the foetal heart.

A diabetic and pregnant woman needs extra 300 kcals per day, the protein content being more. An additional two cups of milk per day should make up the extra demands of 300 kcals. Iron, calcium and vitamin supplements should be taken like other pregnant women. Those who have nausea and loss of appetite in the first three months of pregnancy may have their diet adjusted in this period.

During pregnancy, a diabetic will require diet and either insulin or other oral drugs. Morning sickness may carry a threat of acidosis or insulin reaction. Though serious to the mother, it can be far more dangerous to the unborn child. Hence, as a measure of protection, she needs to take adequate nourishment.

During the second trimester, the placenta produces hormones that will cause changes in your blood sugar, and you may need to increase the dosage of your insulin. Some women may develop diabetes temporarily, known as gestational diabetes, during pregnancy, due to the change in the usual hormone production, and the sugar is not utilised properly. The hormones produced by the placenta block the effect of insulin.

Gestational diabetes is generally treated with diet. When the fasting blood sugar is more than 105 mg per cent, insulin is necessary. If you are able to control the temporary diabetes with diet alone, your pregnancy will be allowed to continue, and you may not need early hospitalisation. If the diabetes found during pregnancy did not exist earlier, it frequently will not be present after delivery. But you do need periodic check-ups as you have an increased risk for developing diabetes later in life.

As an insulin dependent diabetic, you may need double or triple the doses of it as pregnancy progresses. There is nothing to be alarmed about this as this is expected. As your blood sugar increases, there is increased danger of ketoacidosis (diabetic coma), but by frequently testing yourself, you can avoid this state.

During the third semester, your blood and urine are tested for estriol a hormone produced by the foetus and the placenta. The mother and foetus are progressing normally if the estriol levels are within normal ranges. This is done around the 30th week of pregnancy, and then weekly or more often until delivery.

Another ultrasound test is done during this period, and the results compared with the first one, to ensure that the growth of the foetus has progressed satisfactorily, as anticipated. If the growth is not as expected, you may be advised complete bed rest or other changes in your care for the remaining weeks.

Complications in the form of presence of protein in urine and rise in blood pressure are more common in diabetic pregnancy than in a normal pregnancy. If they were existent even before pregnancy, then they may be even higher during pregnancy. Your physician will outline a special programme of daily rest and relaxation for you.

If you have kidney disease, then during pregnancy oedema (retention of water by the tissues of the body) may be aggravated. The amount of fluid in the pregnant uterus is often increased in diabetic pregnancy. The diabetic woman has a greater-than-normal tendency to retain water in her tissues during pregnancy. For this, a low-salt diet is usually important.

There is also the risk of premature labour. Sometimes, it is advisable or necessary to have the baby delivered before it grows too large or dies in the womb during the last weeks of gestation, instead of waiting for the pregnancy to run its full course. The best time would be about three to four weeks before the normal time of birth, and the best person to know this would be your obstetrician.

Certain drugs or other methods can induce normal labour earlier, or the baby may be delivered by Caesarean section. In many cases, hospitalisation just a week before delivery is encouraged. This will help in monitoring carefully your baby's activity and heart rate, and in avoiding last minute difficulties that may arise. During this week, you may undergo the amniocentesis test, a test whereby a sample of amniotic fluid surrounding the foetus will be withdrawn from the uterus. From this sample, measurements of substances produced by the baby's lungs can be taken to determine whether the child's lungs are mature enough for the baby to breathe normally after delivery.

Another complication that may arise, though it is very rare, is eclampsia. This is a serious condition causing convulsions and coma which occurs very rarely during the last three months of child birth. Eclampsia is an advanced stage of what is called toxaemia where there is presence of any poisonous substance in the circulating blood.

A mild degree of toxaemia is fairly common, affecting about one woman in 10 during her first pregnancy, and about one in 20 during later pregnancies. With treatment the condition generally settles down, but a long period of rest in bed may be needed.

There are cases of miscarriages and smaller babies associated with diabetic women who smoke. Smoking affects the growth of the baby and hence should be avoided. Even modest regular alcohol intake in pregnancy will have an unfavourable outcome as far as the baby is concerned. So you should stop drinking alcohol until the pregnancy is over.

Post-delivery Care

Where the diabetes has been well treated, childbirth is more nearly normal. The woman with a good environment usually has an easier time during delivery while many women with diabetes have Caesarean deliveries; there are those who have a vaginal delivery. Caesarean section will also be done if the foetus is in difficulty or is mature enough for birth and labour cannot be induced; or when the mother has retinal disease.

A normal blood glucose level is maintained during labour, preventing the drop of blood glucose level in the newborn. During labour, the insulin requirement may fall, and after delivery falls markedly.

During the first few days after the birth of your baby, you will probably notice a significant decrease in your insulin requirement. Within another few days, you will return to your pre-pregnancy state, and will be able to return to former habits of controlling diabetes. Those with gestational diabetes may become less insulin dependent for an indefinite period, but insulin should not be stopped fully until enough time has lapsed to determine whether the diabetes can be controlled without it.

Your obstetrician will recommend your pre-pregnancy programme of diet, insulin and exercise. If you are nursing your baby, you will need to raise your food intake and may need an insulin dosage adjustment. Breast-feeding is encouraged and your insulin requirements diminish. You should have a snack before nursing the baby.

For a diabetic woman, pregnancy is itself a strain, and since bringing up children is an additional responsibility, she should limit the number of children to the minimum.

The menstrual cycle of diabetic women is often irregular. In such cases, avoid the 'safe period' method of family planning.

Nowadays, with the introduction of low-dose monophasic or triphasic oral contraceptives, the change in insulin and glucose levels are of no significance. In overt diabetic women, the effect on insulin requirement is neither consistent nor predictable, and little, if any, change occurs with low dose pills.

Women with insulin-dependent diabetes mellitus may have the risk of blood clotting. Therefore, they should use other forms of contraception. In women under the age of 35, the risk of blood clotting with low dose oral contraceptive is very minimal, provided they do not smoke, and are healthy.

The chances of developing pelvic infections from intrauterine contraceptive devices are very high if diabetes is uncontrolled.

MENSTRUATION AND MENOPAUSE

Menstruation

Young diabetic women may notice that their menstrual patterns are different from those of women who do not have diabetes. While normal girls begin menstruation between 10 and 14 years of age, some diabetic girls begin as late as 16 years of age, and those whose diabetes is poorly controlled start much later than 16 years. Inappropriate insulin dosage or poor nutrition can cause disturbances of hormonal balance, and thus physical growth.

Irregularity in the monthly cycle is another factor that diabetic women face. Improved control of diabetes will result in increased regularity of the menses.

All women prior to and during menstruation undergo hormonal changes. For the diabetic women, these changes affect how insulin is used, for example, a rise in blood sugar can occur. If you have insulin-dependent diabetes, you may have to re-adjust your insulin dosage, or reduce food intake to negate the possibility of higher blood sugar. During menstruation, your estrogen, progesterone and blood sugar levels will vary. At such times you may be advised to adjust your insulin dosage. You may be put on slight reduction of food intake and fluid intake just before your periods. The kidney threshold for glucose may be reduced during menstruation, and, hence, glucose may appear in urine even with normal blood glucose level.

A diabetic woman is well advised to use sanitary pads instead of tampons, as the latter may give rise to severe bacterial infection that can produce shock. Pelvic infection is more common in tampon users.

Menopause

Menstruation ceases around the age of 40-55 years. Some people cease to have it even earlier. Some stop suddenly, while some have erratic and spaced out menses. Many may think they are now past menstruation, as they have not had one in several months, and then begin menstruating again. This cycle may last from six months to three years. The age at onset is often, but not always, a family trait.

At any age, surgical removal of the ovaries results in an artificial menopause, which occurs abruptly and is often more disturbing than the natural menopause.

A whole train of events starts when egg cells are no longer released from the ovaries, and pregnancy can no longer occur. The ovaries drastically curtail their production of estrogens, menstruation ceases, and the body must adapt to a new hormone balance.

Since all the hormones together control the vital processes in the body, it is natural that a shortage of any of them should temporarily result in some sort of upset. Most women have at least minor physical and physiological disturbances during the time. The most common complaint is hot flushes in which the body temperature suddenly rises and then returns to normal. Other symptoms may include irritability, insomnia, dizziness and depression. The number and severity of the symptoms may vary from woman to woman. A tendency toward brittle bones occurs because of the reduced amount of hormones in the body; many older women sustain fractures because of this change in their bodies.

As an insulin-dependent diabetic woman, you may have some special concerns, like, it may be difficult for you to distinguish menopausal hot flushes from low blood sugar reactions causing similar symptoms. If you feel the hot flushes are from low blood sugar and take extra sugar or food, you may raise your blood sugar too high. And if you consider a hypoglycaemic reaction to be a hot flush, you may neglect to take insulin and make your low blood sugar reaction worse. To avoid this confusion, test your own blood sugar.

If you are 40 years old or more, other symptoms of menopause may also concern you. Your blood sugar level responds to anti-depressive medications as well as to mental stress. To avoid undue stress and the need for anti-depressant medications, proper relaxation and a healthy outlook on life are recommended. Since brittle bones are characteristic of diabetics, particularly in menopausal and post-menopausal women, you may need to supplement your diet with calcium-rich foods.

OTHER SPECIAL PROBLEMS

Insulin Atrophy

This is quite common in women, though rare in adult men. Atrophy is a wasting away or reduction in size of an organ or other parts of the body. In insulin atrophy, the woman whose arms and legs are pitted because of regular insulin injections will be understandably reluctant to wear bathing suits or sleeveless dresses. Insulin atrophy is not as serious physically as it is cosmetically and psychologically. While no cure is yet possible for atrophy, the woman suffering it can certainly find other dress styles to fit her needs.

Fungus Infections

Many disease-producing fungi affect the skin only. Fungus diseases that infect the while system are known as systemic fungus disease, caused by a yeast-like fungus. It is very widespread and has been found in the mouth, vagina and faeces of apparently healthy people. Acute infection is more likely to occur in someone who is affected by diabetes. From young adulthood, it is common among women to have infection in the genital area. It can cause serious itching and discomfort due to an oozing skin eruption. They can be treated with special fungicides and the antibiotic nystatin ointment. Special hygienic care can also help prevent them.

Urinary Infections

Increased frequency in the desire to urinate, generally with only a little urine passed, is often caused by infection. This is more likely in diabetic women in their middle ages. Today, with a wide range of antibiotics at the disposal of the physician, all the infections related to the bladder can be treated.

Heart Ailments

Diabetes seems to increase a woman's susceptibility to heart ailments. Normally, a healthy woman is three times less likely than a man to suffer from heart disease, but diabetes negates this advantage, and makes her equally assailable. People with heart disease should concentrate on eating more of the fibre-rich foods and cut back on fatty foods.

Fertility

In olden days, before the introduction of insulin, conception was a problem with young diabetic women. Now, women with well-controlled diabetes have normal fertility. Extremely poor diabetes control with consistently high blood glucose readings is associated with reduced fertility.

16

DIABETES IN THE YOUNG (BABIES, CHILDREN, ADOLESCENT)

Many parents are deeply affected when their children develop diabetes. It is said that when a child develops diabetes, the doctor immediately has two patients – the child and the mother. The diagnosis of diabetes in a young one frequently sends outs waves of stress which reach far beyond the immediate family – the relatives, other children, friends, and even teachers.

The parents of diabetic child are fraught with emotions, and it is difficult for them to accept it with equanimity. It is no easy matter for the mother to cope with all the day in and day out urine tests, injections, special dieting schedules, programming exercises, eye care, etc. No less is the child troubled. With the help of his parents and physician, the child can learn to live with diabetes in a healthy manner.

DIABETES IN BABIES

Diabetes is very rare in infants less than 12 months old, and so you will not find many paediatricians with experience of this condition. However, the general principles are the same for all infants with diabetes, and there is no reason why the baby should not grow into a healthy young person.

The diabetic baby will be fed on breast or bottle milk. For the first four months, frequent feeds are best three-hourly by day, and four-hourly by night. Bottle-fed babies usually need about 2 ½ ounces (or 37 ml) of milk per ½ kg of weight each day. Some babies grow quite fast and need more milk than this while others may need solids earlier than four months. This benefits babies with diabetes, as the solids will slow down the absorption of milk. It is essential that you wake up the baby for a night feed to avoid night time insulin reactions. To avoid any doubt about this, do a blood glucose check while your baby is asleep. If the blood glucose is low, additional 100-200 ml milk should be given.

It is not easy to get clean samples of urine from babies in nappies. Quite a few produce a little by reflex into a small potty when undressed. Or, you can squeeze a wet nappy directly onto a urine testing stick, but be warned that washing powders or fabric softeners in the nappies alter the urine test result.

Infants are much more likely than older people to have ketones in the urine, because they rapidly switch to burning up fat stores in the fasting state. It is important to check on ketones and try to keep the baby's urine ketone-free, although you should not worry if ketones appear for a short time.

If your baby looks ill or feels unwell, you may have to do a blood test from a finger, heel or earlobe. Urine tests only provide a guide about the state of the baby's diabetes since its last urine test, whereas the blood test confirms what is happening at that very instant. This is the only way to check whether your baby is hypo or just tired and hungry. If the baby's blood glucose rises during an illness, you may have to decide on the dose of insulin, and hence blood glucose measurements are necessary.

As the infant grows up, it needs more solids. Food is of great emotional significance to all children, and all of them go through phases of food refusal. Usually when they begin this phase, at around 8-10 months, they turn their faces away, making feeding impossible. The battle between the baby and mother is even more difficult where the infant has diabetes. You have to find ways to coax the infant to eat at least most of the food, if not all, by distracting it with toys, music, talk, games, etc. Try variations in diet to make it more attractive. You can try biscuits, fruit juices, bread, potatoes, and even ice-creams as alternatives.

If your infant's high glucose level is poorly controlled, chances of shortness in height can result. If you keep his/her diabetes under control, and make sure that he/she has plenty to eat and drink, he/she should grow rapidly, and may gain the natural height. This will also ensure that the infant does not get long-term complications.

DIABETES IN CHILDREN

Parents cannot be expected to accept diabetes in a child casually. But they should help the child by laying emphasis on the child rather than on the disease. They should have a relaxed and calm atmosphere at home, in which both parents play a positive role. The father's role is equally important as it provides an additional measure of stability and security, and gives the child the sense of being cared.

Any child with diabetes can continue to lead a normal childhood, attend school, go to summer camps or tours, travel, and participate in sports. Let your child continue to be a child. With the disease under control, and the child knowledgeable about diabetes, there is nothing to prevent him from participating in strenuous activities.

Diabetes, which is not contagious, is a disorder that rarely goes away by itself. It is important to diagnose it early and start treatment immediately. The aim should be to provide proper growth of the child, both physically and mentally.

The peak incidence of diabetes in children is between five and 15 years of age. Diabetes in children differs from that in adults in several respects.

Causes

The causes of diabetes in young children and adolescents are not known. Heredity does play a role, but it alone is not enough to cause diabetes. Researches reveal that certain viruses may combine with an inherited susceptibility and play a role in the development of diabetes.

An older child will be able to understand all about diabetes, why insulin or tablets are required, the special diet that he needs, etc. Many cases of diabetes under the age of 15 appear suddenly. Unlike non-insulin-dependent diabetes, which is often related to obesity in adults, diabetes in children has little to do with weight. If your child's case is like many of the juvenile diabetic type, it is very likely to be insulin-dependent, and will require daily insulin injections.

The two factors that determine beta cell damage are genetic susceptibility of the host and some environmental factors like viruses, toxins and dietary factors.

Characteristics

Childhood diabetes has some odd features. Once it has been diagnosed and treatment commences, there is frequently a dramatic improvement – the symptoms of diabetes vanish, insulin has to be discontinued, and the child seems to be miraculously cured. But this is just a short phase, and the diabetes flares up again permanently. This is called the honeymoon period. It can be very trying as it raises hopes that the diabetes has cleared up, but, unfortunately, this never happens in young people.

Childhood diabetes is usually of the insulin-dependent type. In children, unlike in adults, the onset of diabetes is usually rapid.

Another characteristic common in all diabetic children until the age of 10 is that an insulin reaction is often accompanied by symptoms that are usually related to the opposite complication — acidosis. These symptoms are vomiting and headache. Never stop the insulin even if your child is vomiting. During feverish illness the body needs more insulin, not less. Even where acidosis is the complication involved, the child who vomits will need sugar along with the insulin. You may have to give three or four injections a day as this is much more flexible, and so the child responds more quickly to changes in the situation. If the child becomes dehydrated in the space of a few hours if vomiting continues, then he will need fluid dripped into a vein, meaning hospitalisation.

Other common features of childhood diabetes are severe thirst, an excessive amount of urine, bed-wetting, weight loss and weakness.

Diet

Each child is different and each child's needs differ from day to day. Children who eat too much may be taking more insulin than they need, and the extra insulin causes increased hunger. However, hunger can also be an indication that the blood sugar is low. A blood test at the time of the child's hunger should tell you exactly whether it is increased blood glucose or genuine hunger. If the blood sugar is often low, you should discuss with the physician about changing the insulin dosage. Adults in whom diabetes sets in later are often overweight, and can be treated with a weight-reduction diet. Not so for a diabetic child for he needs an adequate diet for his growth and physical activities.

Kcal Requirement of Diabetic Child

Age	*Kcal*
3-4	1,300
7-8	1,900
11-12	2,200
17-17	2,400

A rule of thumb is that the kcal requirement of a child is:

1000 + (100 x child's age)

Like all normal children, diabetic ones will also want to snack between meals. An insulin-dependent diabetic child needs to have calculated snacking because the injected insulin continues to work even if no food is eaten: you can give the child a snack if his meal is delayed for some reason, and then the meal should be reduced in size. The recommended snacks for him would be the ones with nutritional value, such as cheese, crackers, skim milk, peanut butter, raisins or other dried fruits.

The requirement of vitamins and minerals of a child with diabetics is the same as that of a healthy child. The protein allowance should be as indicated on the next page.

Protein Allowance for a Diabetic Child

Age	*Daily Protein Allowance gms/ kg (body weight)*
Up to 5	3.5
5 – 7	3.0
7 – 15	2.5
15 – 17	2.0

The child should have regular meal times. He should eat breakfast, lunch, supper, mid-morning snack and bed-time snack containing carbohydrates. This is necessary to avoid hypoglycaemia due to insulin deficiency. The meals of a diabetic child need not be different from that of others, except restrictions on some foodstuffs.

A problem that often springs up is whether a diabetic child should be allowed to have sweets or not. An occasional sweet may be permitted so that he is not tempted to eat it on the sly.

All children love to attend parties, travel, and visit friends overnight. You must then help your child to plan ahead. He may need to consult the doctor on this matter, or you could let the friend's parent provide artificially sweetened ice-cream or beverages for him. He may wish to carry his own refreshments. He should explain to his hostess the need for timing of meals and plan the menu to avoid embarrassment. While a smaller child may need guidance, a teenager generally is able to adjust his own diet.

Most people lose weight before their diabetes is diagnosed and treated. In uncontrolled diabetes body fat is broken down and many calories are lost as glucose in the urine. When the diabetes is brought under control, the body fat stops being broken down, the calories are no longer lost, and the weight loss stops. Many people then begin to put on weight till they reach their original weight.

Insulin in the right dose does not make a child fat, but if he is having too much insulin he will have to eat more to prevent hypos, and these extra calories will increase his weight. When he is on insulin and becomes too fat, then losing extra weight can be a slow business. He cannot afford to have sudden, drastic dieting but can only lose weight by careful reduction of both food and insulin. This can be a delicate balance but many people manage it successfully. Hence, it is better to avoid putting on weight in the first place.

There is this risk of weight gain when children stop growing. When they are growing tall, they do need enormous quantities of food, but once their growth is complete they need to make dietary changes by reducing their total food intake. Girls usually stop growing a year or two after menses sets in, and unless they eat a lot less, at this stage they will most certainly become fat, and then shedding off excess weight becomes difficult.

Insulin

The administration of insulin may be one of the most important problems at the outset. A child might be frightened of the pain and the appearance of a hypodermic syringe.

The parent should try to keep the insulin injection simple and easy to handle. The syringe should be prepared and the dose measured out of the child's sight initially. Then the injection should be given without any fuss.

Initially the child can have the injections on the buttocks, which are less sensitive to pain. Do not set a precedent of cajoling or bribing the child to have his injections, neither should you scold or threaten him, but try to make him understand the importance of it. If the child has a normally good adjustment, the injection will not create too great a problem. Whatever the circumstance, the insulin injection must be given in the proper dosage at the proper time.

As the child grows older, changes in living patterns bring inevitable changes in the problems of treatment. The child begins to go to bed later, he stays out and plays longer. These and similar developments are sure to demand changes and adjustments in the insulin as well in the eating schedule.

Diabetic children are insulin-dependent, and oral drugs are useless for them. When some infection sets in or the blood glucose level is very high, the child may need a short-acting insulin three or four times a day.

In the beginning, an experienced person should inject insulin, and gradually the child can inject himself, after some encouragement and instructions. The parents should supervise every now and then the child's method of injecting himself.

Exercise

Children get a lot of exercise during playtime, running and jumping. They often participate in vigorous activities such as football, tennis, bicycling, etc. Exercise, a natural part of childhood, is essential to control diabetes, as the child burns up sugar, thus decreasing his need of insulin. He has less chances of becoming overweight, and his blood circulation too will improve. The physician may recommend extra food for needed energy or special snacks before a game to avoid low blood sugar. He may also change the dose of insulin to allow for the extra exercise.

Due to the extreme instability of juvenile diabetes, many seemingly ordinary things, such as the season of the year, weather and temperature, may cause problems, affecting the child's need for insulin. On a bright, sunny day, playing outside the home may reduce his need for insulin. On a rainy day, his physical activity is reduced, thereby causing an increase in insulin need.

Hypoglycaemia

A child in hypo may become unusually quiet, inattentive, morose, or irritable. At night, a hypo may cause a headache, and in the morning lead to fatigue.

Parents, teachers and close friends should know the warning symptoms of hypoglycaemia so that immediate treatment can be given to the child. It is very important for the child to carry some glucose, and take it dissolved in water when the warning signals set in. He should also always carry with him an identity card.

As the physical activities of a child are erratic, it is better to give him snacks during a burst of activities rather than reduce the dose of insulin.

When there is low blood glucose at night, it can give rise to an increase in blood glucose level with glucose in urine the next morning. It is important to recognise this strangely paradoxical increase in the morning blood glucose level, and accordingly reduce the dose of evening intermediate acting insulin.

Many teenagers overeat to avoid a hypo, but it is important to explain to them the need for spacing the meals and snacks in between the meals, and the repercussions of overeating.

Urine Test

Due to the diabetic child's high sensitivity to insulin, a sugar-free urine may lead to frequent incidents of insulin reaction. So some urinary sugar is permissible at various times during the day. A child's control of his diabetes is usually good if the morning test shows no sign of urinary acetone.

Around the age of 9 to 11, many diabetic children can manage their own insulin injections and urine testing. Some may prefer to monitor blood sugar levels instead of urine test. This would be better as blood tests give a clearer picture control, for they give exact measures of blood sugar.

Home Blood Glucose Monitoring

Whenever possible, home blood glucose monitoring should be done to have good control over diabetes throughout the day, to adjust the balance of insulin, diet and exercise. It is also useful in checking whether you have hypoglycaemia.

School Schedules

It is always better to let the school personnel know about your child's daily plan for balancing diet and insulin, and provide them with information about the child's daily dietary requirements. For example, the teacher should know that the child has to have a mid-morning snack, and it could be during class hours. He should be allowed to spend five minutes or so to eat it, and the child should not be punished for doing so, or refused to allow eating his snacks.

Since the child faces special challenges in the school setting, probably being the only child to be receiving insulin, special diet, etc., at the beginning of the academic year, the parents should meet the class teacher and discuss with him the needs of the child, for instance, timely meals, timely snacks, physical activities, precautions while he is having a hypo, etc.

Children who have to test urine or blood for sugar level before lunch should be allowed to leave the classroom for this purpose. Many children usually need a small dose of quick-acting insulin along with a large dose of slower, longer-acting insulin. The regular insulin acts only in the four hours between breakfast and lunch. The long-acting insulin works for the rest of the day. Regular insulin should also be reduced if he has frequent insulin reactions between breakfast and lunch. On the other hand, if he spills sugar or passes urine frequently during that period, regular insulin should be increased.

If the school schedule delays the child's lunch, a reduction in the regular insulin may be necessary to avoid the possibility of insulin reaction. Similarly, eating schedules can also be modified to meet the needs of living. If he normally takes his lunch around moon, and the school lunch hour interval is at 1 pm, he may need to have more snacks during his mid-morning intake.

It would be wiser for your child to carry his lunch from home instead of eating in a school canteen, where he might get high-carbohydrate meals only. While normally nourishing, these represent a certain amount of wasted eating for the child who cannot utilise certain carbohydrates as well as other children. He can take some high protein foods such as meats, fish, eggs or cheese from home, which he can use without waste.

Your child's friends may suddenly spot a man outside the school selling ice-creams. Soon they will all be eating ice-cream, but your child will have to exercise self-discipline and refuse to share in the fun. Not that he cannot have them, he can, but only at certain stipulated times within his schedule, while the others can have them any time, and as often as they wish.

Emotional Problems

Some children, especially the older ones, are emotionally disturbed when they realise that they have diabetes for life. Faced with daily doses of injections, blood glucose and urine tests, diet restrictions and schedules, etc., the child's hurt mind takes some time to come to grips with reality and the way of things to come. He knows that he has to make certain adjustments, and the parents, teachers, friends and relatives need to give him a supporting hand at this time. But once he comes to terms with the situation, he finds that he can be like other children with just a few restrictions, and still lead a healthy life.

It is very important that your child tells his close friends that he has diabetes. He should explain about hypos and tell that if he does behave in an odd way they should make him take sugar and he should show them where he keeps his supplies. If your child shows his friends how he measures his blood glucose they will most certainly be interested in diabetes, and be eager to help him with it. As he becomes older and spends more time away from home he will come to depend more on his friends. For any child, though, this will be a traumatic experience, but the stronger his sense of security, the better he usually weathers it.

The family's support plays a vast role in stabilising the child's emotionally traumatic state. Sparks of rebellion and non-cooperation are bound to show up every now and then, especially as he approaches adolescence. But these outbursts usually die down with the helpful and understanding attitude of his parents and siblings.

Both over-indulgence and neglect, while they do damage to the child, are rooted in the personality and adjustment problems of the parents. To rectify or correct them, intelligence and human understanding are more important than medical understanding. But rapid restriction of a child often can be corrected by improved medical understanding.

As the diabetic child grows older and he shows signs of resentment and rebellion, he will discover that his urine tests do not immediately show a rise in sugar even if he takes a forbidden chocolate or eats a helping of ice-cream on the quiet. At other times, his sugar may rise even though he has kept strictly to his diet. All this makes him question the validity of the restrictions. He may then begin to violate them, trying to follow what other normal children are permitted to do.

If the parent-child relationship is a good one, this rebellion should not get out of control, and will probably be amenable to adjustment. If the relationship is a bad one, or the treatment has been too rigid, the rebellion could persist with serious consequences.

In the normal process of growing up, revolt against authority is a common occurrence. In the diabetic child, it has an additional spur. The intelligent parent must understand this, anticipate it and be prepared to compensate for it with additional insulin or whatever else might be indicated.

About the best that can be hoped for is to have the rebellion minimised and kept within bounds. This goal can best be attained where the family relationships are good and where the treatment is balanced between the needs of the ailment and the human needs of the child.

Overprotection of the child hinders his psychological development. The child should not be allowed to use diabetes as a means to escape unpleasant situations like school examinations. Too much affection and attention on the diabetic child may lead to the feeling among the other children in the family of being neglected.

A diabetic teenager often develops anxiety about the future career, job or marriage and needs proper counselling. With proper understanding and right attitudes, a diabetic child can mature normally, physically and psychologically.

In childhood, there is also a flood of birthday parties, becoming more numerous as the child's circle of friends expands. At these parties there is the usual gorging of ice-cream, chocolates, cakes, potato chips, etc., washed down by various kinds of soda pop. While others are stuffing themselves with all the goodies, the diabetic child must not indulge in.

If the party is timed to coincide with the child's snack time, the parent can make adjustments so that the child could have an ice-cream or some other item that is normally not allowed for him. This may ease the situation, but there is no getting away from the fact that it will not entirely remove the mounting sense of 'difference'.

Summer Camps and School Trips

Recently, summer camps for diabetic children have begun in India. Here the children meet other children with diabetes who too are learning to cope with the disease. These camps are of great value in teaching children to live with diabetes. There is a good gathering of doctors, nurses and dieticians along with diabetic children.

Beside the usual recreational activities of the camp, the children are taught how to test urine, how to monitor home blood glucose, the technique of injecting insulin, diet schedules and the importance of exercises. These activities help the children to become self-reliant and be able to cope with the disease successfully.

Your child should carry with him a travel kit for storing his supplies of insulin, tablets and other necessary items. A doctor's prescription should also be handy in case the child runs out of medicines, or syringe, etc., and in case of emergency, the teacher in the camp can give him insulin injection or glucose, so that child should also have glucose available, and he can carry some necessary snacks like biscuits, cheese, etc.

Your child should continue to test his glucose routinely, just as he would at home. He also needs to have scheduled timings for his meals and snacks, and the teachers should be apprised of this.

In some of the special camps for diabetic children, during the rainy weather, the children exercise indoors on treadmills to obtain the physical activity they would otherwise miss. These camps also provide healthful recreation and a wide variety of sports activities.

When a child finds it difficult to adjust to his diabetes in the initial years, if he feels isolated or unique, if he seems overly dependent in handling his urine and blood glucose tests and other chores, then a diabetic camp might be very useful. For a child with a good attitude toward his disease, he would be better off in a regular camp with his everyday friends when he would learn, as he must, to function in a non-diabetic world.

School trips can also be useful and recreating. Day trips should be no problem as long as someone can be sure that he eats on time, and has his second injection if necessary.

At the junior level, long trips away from home could be more difficult, and it really depends on you finding a member of staff who you can trust to take care of him. They will need to keep an eye on your child and to know how to cope sensibly with problems like bad hypo. Once in the secondary or high school, most children manage to go away on trips with the school, scout or a youth group. Needless to say, one of the adults in the party should be responsible, but as your child gets older he will be able to look after himself.

Coping with a Diabetic Child

Apart from general rules, there are some specific suggestions, which will help parents and the child to achieve a better adjustment to the disease. As you learn to help your child regulate his body chemistry for a healthier life, remember to do what your physician advises. You will become intelligently informed about diabetes and seek out the latest scientific information. Friends and relatives will offer well-meaning advice and suggestions that may not be applicable to your child. Some of these advices may just be mumbo-jumbo and old wives' tales. So be prudent and follow your doctor's instructions.

Control of your child's diabetes will depend on proper diet, emotional stability, well-regulated insulin injections, exercise, and regular glucose testing.

You should avoid bribing, cajoling or intimidating your child to accept insulin injections and other necessities of treatment. While you accept the fact, try to have the child accept the fact that the insulin injections, while painful, are necessary. The same applies to such deprivations as denial of certain foods and activities.

Families that have adjusted well to caring for a diabetic child do not make the child's diabetes a central concern to the family and do not need to change the entire family's lifestyle. You should try to treat the disease in such a way that it seems to cause the least visible disruption in everyday living. The regular living habits of the family should go on as before. The other children should be treated exactly the same as before, allowed to eat the same, play the same, have the same right. If you set reasonable goals for diet, testing, exercise, and self-care, your child will adapt to the situation with flexibility and good humour, and so will others in the family.

By following these suggestions it would be possible for you to establish a situation in which a diabetic child has a maximum feeling of security as an individual and as a member of the family. The closer this situation is achieved, the better will be the child's attitude toward his disease, and the fewer will be the strains set up within the family.

The best help you can give your child with diabetes is to keep calm and not show constant concern over every detail of the management of the disease. Your practical attitude will rule off on your child. If you accept the extra activities of daily living related to diabetic care as part of the family routine, so will your child, who will soon come to see diabetes as an uncomplicating aspect of life.

If your child takes insulin shots, he will learn to cope with the minor discomfort as part of his routine, just as he accepts daily hygiene routines, occasional falls, grazed knees, and other cuts and bruises. If you express too much sympathy for occasional discomfort, or fuss too much over it, your child may begin to feel sorry for him, and thus have a harder time taking the injections and caring for himself.

You should ensure that your child does not use diabetes as an excuse for avoiding special lessons, or necessary activities that he may not enjoy. He may, of course, have occasional headache, or stomach pain, or a sick spell, like any normal child. However, you should encourage him to view these things as something to overcome, not something to hide behind. By not being over-protective, and by encouraging your child to carry on routine activities in spite of some occasional setbacks, your child will develop a mature outlook toward living with diabetes. Overall, your role in coping with your diabetic child will be supportive but should not be over-indulgent. Try to encourage self-care and participations in routine activities.

At times you may suspect that hypoglycaemia is taking place in your child. Use a self-monitoring blood glucose test, or use a urine test for acetone, a sign of possible ketoacidosis (diabetic coma). Ketones do not always indicate ketoacidosis, as it may result from emotional stress, diet, exercise and especially low blood sugar.

DIABETES IN ADOLESCENTS

People vary very greatly in their mental response to developing diabetes. Some lucky one takes to their new condition easily, while others find the whole thing depressing. The depression seems to take two forms. At first, there is shock and even anger at the very onset coupled with fear of injections and the unspoken fear of complications. A few days later come the depressing realisation that diabetes is for life, and not just a temporary disease that can be cured. This type of depression seems to affect the young adolescents who are worried and are feeing insecure about the future.

Since adolescence is a time of great change and upheaval, diabetes developed in the period is the juvenile form with its explosive onset and tendency toward ketosis.

Insulin and Diet

A diabetic adolescent has problems imposed by diabetes compounded by all the other growing up problems that teenagers face. Against the background of these new complexities, the care of adolescent diabetes becomes much more difficult than childhood diabetes.

What seems a frightening thing to most parents is that there is a steep rise in the need for insulin. Daily requirements of 80 to 100 units are common. This is perfectly normal within the framework of diabetes. Later, as the adolescent becomes an adult, the need for insulin will generally decline.

The reason why adolescents need more insulin than children and adults are related to two factors – calories and hormones.

The metabolic activity is greater in adolescence than at any other time. The demand for calories is greater during growth. In his late teens, a boy needs about 4,000 calories daily, almost twice what he will need as an adult. Most of these calories are taken in the form of carbohydrates, like cereals, bread, potatoes, as well as fruits, ice-cream, cake and puddings. This in itself results in a sharp use in the need for insulin.

There is a tendency for an adolescent to spill more sugar into his urine despite the increased insulin. This is perfectly normal for there is a huge consumption of carbohydrate. Hence, this need not worry you too much, so long as your son/daughter is growing well and shows none of the other diabetes symptoms.

The other reason for the big need for insulin is hormones. As the teenager grows, his endocrine activities rise and more hormones are produced and poured into the blood – hormones of the pituitary, thyroid and adrenal glands. These hormones tend to inhibit the activity of insulin, and therefore, more is needed to make up for the reduced efficiency.

Parental supervision will play a role in consumption of alcoholic beverages. Parents may wish to make their own family habits regarding this matter known to the child's physician. In some cases, alcohol can have serious consequences, especially for an insulin-dependent diabetic. In a non-insulin-dependent diabetic who takes one of the oral hypoglycemic, alcohol may cause extreme flushing, and one may notice a very warm sensation and some redness of the skin. But if one's diabetes is out of control, consumption of alcoholic beverages should be totally avoided.

If your son is on insulin, he must be aware of some problems that alcohol can cause; in particular it can make hypos more serious. In such a case, a number of hormones are produced which make the liver release glucose into the bloodstream. As little as two pints of beer will disallow the liver from releasing glucose, and hypos will be more sudden and more severe.

The overall effect of a particular drink depends on the proportions of alcohol to carbohydrate. Your son may notice that beer will have a different effect on blood glucose from vodka. If he has taken alcoholic drinks in the evening, his blood glucose may drop in the early hours of the morning. To counteract this it would be sensible for him to eat a sandwich or something similar, which has long-lasting carbohydrates, before going to bed.

The best way for your son is to find out how an alcohol affects him is for him to have it at home, and measure his blood glucose every hour. This will show him how different quantities of drink affect him. Some people are sometimes accused of being drunk when really they have become hypo after a modest dose of alcohol.

Ideally it would be better if your son could try not to have more than two three units of alcohol in any one session, that is, one unit is half a pint of beer or one glass of wine or one measure of brandy/whiskey, etc. If he is going to have more than this amount, make sure he has his usual meal before he goes out, has a snack while out, and very importantly, has a sandwich before going to bed.

Menstruation and Puberty

Endocrine changes that come with puberty sometimes impose additional problem with girls. In spite of the overall rise in insulin need, menstruation may make an even further demand. The teenage girl may find that she needs a larger dose of insulin a couple of days before the onset of her period. This increased dose will have to be there till about the second day of her period after which it can usually be brought back to normal. The phase of the rise and fall of insulin need associated with the menstrual cycle may go on till menopause.

Adolescent girls frequently refuse to take any urine tests during menstruation. At such times the wise counsel of the physician and the parents must prevail. It is essential to have urine tests for adolescent diabetes, and this must not be discontinued for any reason.

A major upset to the system such as diabetes may cause periods to stop in a young girl. They do mostly reappear within two years if her diabetes is well controlled and she is not underweight.

On average, girls with diabetes do tend to begin their menstruation at an older age. An overweight diabetic girl needs to reduce her intake of food and probably have an adjustment in her insulin dosage.

Adolescence is a time when the activity of the endocrine glands is at its peak. The dynamic changes begun at puberty rise to a crescendo and invoke the pituitary, the thyroid, the adrenal, and other glands.

If your son is sexually underdeveloped even at the age of 16 years or so, then he will certainly have a growth spurt when he goes into puberty. If he remains short or undersized, it could be poor diabetes control that has stunted his growth. But there are other possible factors, including the physical stature of his parents.

Exercise and Self-care

Adolescent girls become increasingly sedentary while boys become more active. Hence, the risk of accident and injury is more likely among boys. Despite this, they should be encouraged to participate in sports and other physical activities. Parents should not try to have diabetic children excused from gymnasium and athletic events. For the teenager, childhood infections are no longer a problem. Colds and accidents though are problems, they are not serious ones, and they enjoy outside activities.

It is essential that adolescents be allowed to engage in normal activities for it will boost their morale and sense of social status, as also self-confidence. But they must remember to have a chocolate or drink juice before a game.

Diabetic teenagers should be allowed to run, jump, play baseball, cricket, football, hockey, basketball or badminton. Even a gruelling game of tennis may be allowed provided they take their insulin shots, and snack before and after the game. If the game continues to be a long-drawn one, then the child should be allowed to have a sustaining drink.

All other normal activities should also be encouraged. The diabetic adolescents, like their normal counterparts, can stay out late, or spend the night with a friend, or even take a vacation away from home. All that is needed is proper provision for the urine tests and insulin injections.

A few people with diabetes feel that, in some way, they are imperfect, especially if previously they have been fitness fanatics. The best way to get round this feeling of inadequacy is to throw themselves into sporting activities with extra enthusiasm. Exercise is good for all of us, and people with diabetes have managed to reach the top in most forms of sports. By treating their diabetes in a positive way rather than letting the condition control them, their depression will gradually clear away.

The full responsibility for all phases of control must rest with the diabetic adolescent, and parents should understand this. They must yield completely all of the daily chores relating to the disease. If this is not done, the teenager may become overly dependent and unable to face the problems of adulthood. Or else the revolt may either take a more serious turn or he may fail to mature properly. If the parents suspect the child's ability to handle the disease and try to control indirectly or secretly, the child is bound to sense it and may lose his grip on his self-confidence.

Stress causes a release of adrenaline and other hormones which antogonise the effect of insulin. In general, stress and worry tend to increase the blood glucose, especially during the run up to the final examination. At such times your child should double his/her insulin dose to keep perfect health.

During stressful times it may be difficult to strictly adhere to meal times. So your child could be going hypo. He then needs to check his blood glucose, and if it not below normal, then he is simply experiencing the tiredness we all feel after studying hard. Instead of blaming it on his diabetes, he should have an evening off from his studies.

Emotional Problems

Emotionally, the adolescent swings between childhood and adulthood erratically. There is great instability, touchiness and sensitivity as his personality seeks to adjust it. He may feel constrained by the controls imposed upon him, and may feel resentful and rebellious. He tries to assert himself and make his own decisions regarding himself and his life by casting off parental control.

The teenager experiences great conflicts both within himself and with his environment. He is more fervid about his rights and independence than the child or adult.

The impact of social and emotional problems upon diabetes is greater in adolescence than at any other time of life. And diabetes has an equally disturbing effect upon the social and emotional adjustments of the adolescent. He often uses his diabetes as a weapon of rebellion against his parents in order to assert himself. He may become lax in taking insulin at the right times, and may suddenly resist the testing of urine. Or he may go on an overnight date and delay the morning injection until he returns home.

Parents should realise that defiance or rebellion is a normal stage of adolescence whether or not diabetes is involved. They should give some leeway to him instead of imposing rigid restrictions, and be tolerant and understanding.

Though the situation with boys is bad, it is definitely worse where the diabetic is a girl. As she is intensely conscious of her competition with other girls for the attention of boys and possible husbands, diabetes presents a tremendous handicap, which, she feels, needs to be kept a secret. She would resent her parents divulging such a guarded secret even to her best friend. Hence, parents, realising secrecy is important to many adolescents during a stage of growing up, must respect their wishes. The best and most intelligent thing they can do, with assistance from the physician, is to teach the adolescent the importance of letting someone in the circle of friends know about the disease. The choice of who is to be informed must be left to the diabetic.

Another problem that the parents have may be lack of communication with their child. The child goes to school and spends more and more time away from home as he or she seeks to form a living pattern of his or her own. This normally brings anxious moments to parents, which is compounded if their child is diabetic. At such a time the understanding parents should never try to force trust and communication, but can be supportive and tolerant.

A diabetic girl is specially prone to fear the future and anticipate all sorts of hardships and obstacles in the way of a normal life. She may feel that diabetes may interfere with her normal physical development or menstrual cycle, that it will interfere with her marriage, and may rule out motherhood. All these fears are groundless. It depends on the individual and the world around her. To tell or not tell would be one of the thorniest problems facing her when she goes out with her boyfriend. It would be better for her to tell him at the beginning. Instead of broadcasting the fact, she can drop a few hints about it, perhaps during a meal together. If the relationship grows, they will want to share each other's problems, including diabetes.

Then there is the question of whether your child can smoke. Smoking is unhealthy not only because it causes cancer of the lung, but because it leads to hardening of the arteries. Hence, the proper advice to all people, especially teenagers, is not to smoke. Smoking will not directly affect the diabetes, except perhaps by reducing appetite. But better to be safe than always be at risk of complications.

Engagement and Marriage

If you want to keep your diabetes a secret from your boyfriend, no major issues are involved so long as it is a platonic relationship. But if the dating turns into courtship, then you do need to reveal your secret about your diabetes. The question is—when? If you have a wholesome attitude to the disease and with no feeling of inferiority, you will probably tell about it at the beginning of the courtship. If you are less secure, you will wait, and then be torn by a sense of guilt. You will probably wait for your engagement before revealing it to your fiancée.

Each diabetic will react in his own individual way, and hence there can be no advice. The insecure diabetic may tell when the guilt overbalances the insecurity. One point can validly be made. If the courtship or engagement were to break up over the matter of diabetes, the overwhelming possibility is that the relationship did not have a sound foundation to start with. In a good relationship, such a matter would be of least concern, for diabetes is not a barrier to marriage.

The percentage of marriages among diabetics is about the same as among non-diabetics. Some diabetics have no problems with their marriage; some have disappointing episodes, with diabetes used as an excuse.

With modern-day management of diabetes, there is every reason for the diabetic boy or girl to approach the possibility of marriage secure in the knowledge that he or she will be every bit as good a partner as the non-diabetic, physically, emotionally, socially, and intellectually.

Impotence

Impotence is common in non-diabetic as well as diabetic men. It is the inability of a man to complete sexual intercourse. Although the term is sometimes taken to mean the same as sterility, technically the two conditions are different. A sterile man cannot produce any or enough healthy sperm cells to become a father; but he can have intercourse. An impotent man may produce sperm cells, but is unable to have an erection and perform sexual intercourse.

Impotence may have a physical or an emotional cause. On the physical side, there may be a defect in the sex organs, a deficiency of the thyroid or pituitary gland, a chronic disease such as anaemia or diabetes, or addiction to alcohol or drugs.

Impotence worries many people and is certainly not so rare that we can ignore it. It is believed that many males at some stage become impotent. Any non-diabetic person may find that he is temporarily impotent, and there is no reason why men with diabetes should not also experience this. Fear of failure can perpetuate this condition. Worry or stress or overwork may be the cause of lack of interest in sex and even of impotence. Excess alcohol can cause prolonged lack of potency.

Some men with diabetes do fall prey to impotency, due to problems with the blood or nerve supply to the penis. This normally sets in gradually, and in the younger person it can be prevented by strict blood glucose control. In the older person the condition does not usually respond well to treatment.

Depending on the cause of impotency, there are several forms of therapy that are effective. Testosterone is effective in those with a hormone deficiency. Vacuum therapy, injections of papaverine and penile implants are effective measures.

Careers

Diabetes does not impair the intelligence and has no effect on the ability to learn. There is no restriction upon diabetes in college or professional schools. They can become engineers, lawyers, nurses, doctors, businessmen, administrators, scientists, etc., but military service is closed to diabetics.

The young diabetic should realise that certain fields of jobs are blocked, like teaching, police, fire department, and pilots of commercial aircraft or ship's officers. The reason is the possibility of insulin shock, which, at a critical moment, might endanger the passenger. While practically all of the professions and most of the jobs will be open to him, he should avoid accepting a job which may create a hazard to him or shock. His diabetes will have no appreciable effect upon his ability to compete with other young men or women for an education and a career.

If you are employed, you should warn fellow employees that you are subject to hypos, so that in case of an emergency, they know what is to be done on the spot.

17

DIABETES AND THE HEART

The heart is a muscular pump that transports blood throughout the body. Together, the heart and blood vessels compose the cardiovascular system. In the general population, the risk of disorders affecting the heart and cardiovascular system increases with age.

This process, which involves the buildup of plaque (atherosclerosis) within artery walls, occurs at a faster rate in patients with diabetes. High levels of glucose (blood sugar) damage the arteries, making them lose their elasticity and causing them to narrow. As a result, blood pressure increases, placing further strain on blood vessels and organs throughout the body.

When this process occurs within the coronary arteries that serve the heart, the condition is called coronary artery disease (CAD). Patients with diabetes are two to four times more likely to develop CAD than nondiabetics, according to the U.S. Centers for Disease Control and Prevention (CDC). Furthermore, the type of plaque that develops in people with diabetes may be more dangerous.

Plaque is a mixture of fats (lipids) and other substances covered by a calcified cap. In patients with diabetes, this cap is thin and vulnerable to rupture by the rushing blood, particularly if the patient has high blood pressure. If this cap is

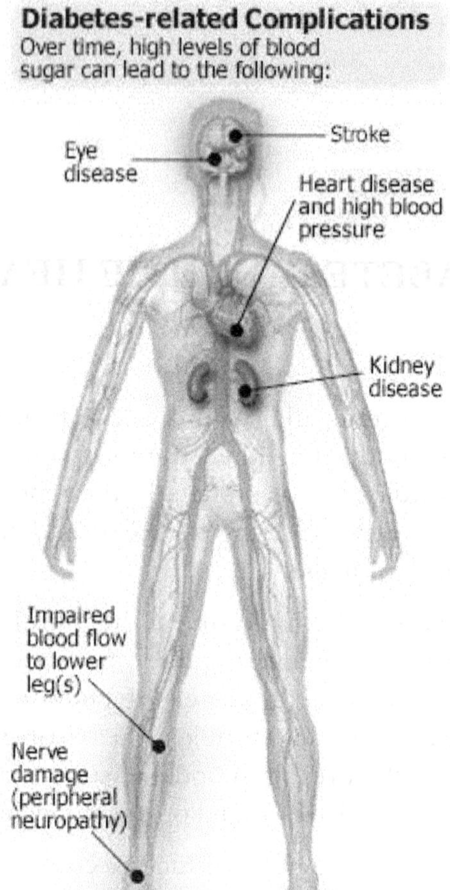

shorn off, the fatty core within is exposed to the bloodstream, which can cause it to clot over again and further obstruct the blood vessel. In addition, pieces of plaque can travel to other vulnerable arteries, blocking them as well.

A heart attack (myocardial infarction) occurs when a coronary artery becomes blocked and heart tissue dies from lack of blood. Depending on the severity of the attack, the heart muscle may become seriously weakened (a condition called cardiomyopathy) and may eventually begin to fail, a condition called heart failure.

Cardiovascular diseases are the primary cause of premature death in patients with diabetes. At least 65 percent of people with diabetes die from heart disease or stroke, according to the CDC. The impact of diabetes on the heart has been compared to surviving a first heart attack among nondiabetics, because the risk of a second, possibly fatal, heart attack is that much greater.

These risks exist for people with either type 1 or type 2 diabetes. However, many of the risk factors for developing type 2 diabetes and related complications (e.g., obesity, high blood pressure and high cholesterol) are also the same for heart disease.

The CDC in 2006 reported that three of the four primary risk factors for cardiovascular disease—high blood pressure, hyperlipidemia and smoking - declined dramatically in prevalence over the past three decades. However, the other one—diabetes - became more common.

Although type 1 diabetes cannot be prevented, patients who have elevated glucose levels but not yet type 2 diabetes (a condition called prediabetes) may be able to prevent or delay diabetes as well as heart disease.

People with lesser-known forms of diabetes, such as maturity-onset diabetes of the young (MODY) and latent autoimmune diabetes of adulthood (LADA), also face increased cardiovascular risks. Prediabetes has also been found to contribute to heart problems. Recent research indicates that prediabetic levels of hyperglycemia contribute to millions of deaths annually from cardiovascular disease. In addition, metabolic syndrome, a cluster of conditions that often include prediabetes, predisposes individuals to heart conditions.

18

DIABETES AND HYPERTENSION

High blood pressure (hypertension) is a sign that the heart and blood vessels are being overworked. The condition is a major factor in the health complications that occur in people with diabetes, and controlling blood pressure is crucial to maintaining good health.

High blood pressure occurs when the force of blood against artery walls becomes excessive. In people with diabetes, high blood pressure increases the risk of serious and life-threatening diseases, including:

- Vascular damage (diabetic angiopathy and atherosclerosis)
- Heart attack, other heart conditions and stroke
- Diabetic nephropathy and chronic kidney failure
- Eye diseases such as diabetic retinopathy and glaucoma

Most people with diabetes have or will develop high blood pressure. Because diabetes and high blood pressure are so closely linked, the American College of Physicians emphasizes that controlling blood pressure should be as high a priority for people with diabetes as controlling glucose (blood sugar).

In addition, people with diabetes are classified as hypertensive earlier than nondiabetics. Nondiabetics are

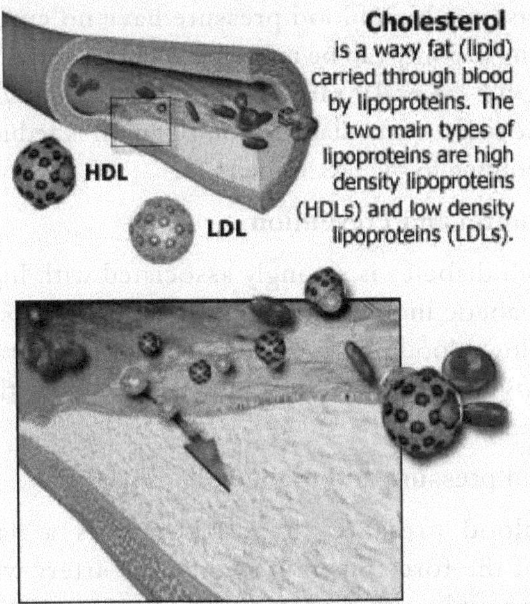

HDLs (good cholesterol) carry LDLs (bad cholesterol) away from artery walls. LDLs stick to artery walls and can lead to plaque build-up (atherosclerosis).

considered to be hypertensive when their blood pressure measures 140/90 millimeters of mercury (mmHg) or higher. Blood pressure is considered high when either the top number (systolic pressure) or the bottom number (diastolic pressure) is above those levels. People with diabetes are classified as hypertensive when systolic pressure is 130 mmHg or higher, or diastolic pressure is 80 mmHg or higher.

The American Diabetes Association (ADA) and the National Heart, Lung and Blood Institute recommend that patients with diabetes and/or kidney disease receive treatment if their blood pressure is above 130/80 mmHg. These levels are slightly stricter than those recommended for the general population.

The ADA recommends that people with diabetes have their blood pressure checked during every visit to a physician, or at least two to four times each year.

Most cases of high blood pressure have no cure, but the overwhelming majority can be managed with diet and medication. In general, for every 10 mmHg reduction in systolic blood pressure, the risk for any diabetic complication is reduced by 12 percent, according to the U.S. Centers for

Disease Control and Prevention

Although diabetes is strongly associated with high blood pressure, diabetic individuals can also experience potentially dangerous low blood pressure (hypotension). Several factors linked to this condition can be addressed to reduce the risk of dizziness and fainting.

About blood pressure and diabetes

High blood pressure (hypertension) is a dangerous elevation of the force pushing against the artery walls. It is common in people with diabetes.

Between 60 and 65 percent of people with diabetes have high blood pressure, according to the National Institute of Diabetes and Digestive and Kidney Diseases (NIDDK). The National Diabetes Education Program raises that estimate to 70 percent. African Americans, American Indians and Alaska Natives are particularly at risk.

19

DIABETIC EYE PROBLEMS

Also called: Diabetic retinopathy

Do you know what causes the most blindness in U.S. adults? It is an eye problem caused by diabetes, called diabetic retinopathy. Your retina is the light-sensitive tissue at the back of your eye. You need a healthy retina to see clearly.

Diabetic retinopathy happens when diabetes damages the tiny blood vessels inside your retina. You may not notice at first. Symptoms can include

- Blurry or double vision
- Rings, flashing lights or blank spots
- Dark or floating spots
- Pain or pressure in one or both of your eyes
- Trouble seeing things out of the corners of your eyes

If you have diabetes, you should have a complete eye exam every year. Finding and treating problems early may save your vision. Treatment often includes laser treatment or surgery.

What can I do to prevent diabetes eye problems?

- Keep your blood glucose and blood pressure as close to normal as you can.

- Have an eye care professional examine your eyes once a year. Have this exam even if your vision is OK. The eye care professional will use drops to make the black part of your eyes-pupils-bigger. This process is called dilating (DY-layt-ing) your pupil, which allows the eye care professional to see the back of your eye. Finding eye problems early and getting treatment right away will help prevent more serious problems later on.

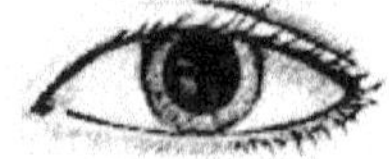

Dilated eye

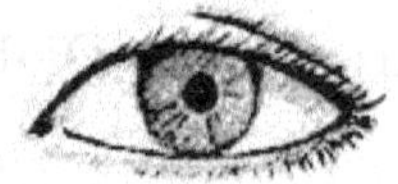

Undilated eye

- Ask your eye care professional to check for signs of cataracts and glaucoma. (See What other eye problems can diabetes cause? to learn more about cataracts and glaucoma.)
- If you are pregnant and have diabetes, see an eye care professional during your first 3 months.
- If you are planning to get pregnant, ask your doctor if you should have an eye exam.
- Don't smoke.

How can diabetes hurt my eyes?

High blood glucose and high blood pressure from diabetes can hurt four parts of your eye:

1. Retina (RET-ih-nuh). The retina is the lining at the back of the eye. The retina's job is to sense light coming into the eye.
2. Vitreous (VIT-ree-uhss). The vitreous is a jelly-like

fluid that fills the back of the eye.

3. Lens. The lens is at the front of the eye. It focuses light on the retina.
4. Optic nerve. The optic nerve is the eye's main nerve to the brain.

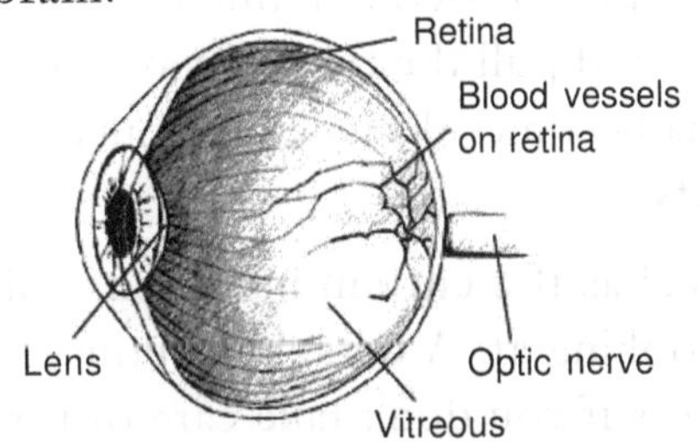

This is a picture of an eye from the side.

How can diabetes hurt the retinas of my eyes?

Retina damage happens slowly. Your retinas have tiny blood vessels that are easy to damage. Having high blood glucose and high blood pressure for a long time can damage these tiny blood vessels.

First, these tiny blood vessels swell and weaken. Some blood vessels then become clogged and do not let enough blood through. At first, you might not have any loss of sight from these changes. Have a dilated eye exam once a year even if your sight seems fine.

One of your eyes may be damaged more than the other. Or both eyes may have the same amount of damage.

Diabetic retinopathy (RET-ih-NOP-uh-thee) is the medical term for the most common diabetes eye problem.

What happens as diabetes retina problems get worse?

As diabetes retina problems get worse, new blood vessels grow. These new blood vessels are weak. They break easily and leak blood into the vitreous of your eye. The leaking blood keeps light from reaching the retina.

You may see floating spots or almost total darkness. Sometimes the blood will clear out by itself. But you might need surgery to remove it.

Over the years, the swollen and weak blood vessels can form scar tissue and pull the retina away from the back of the eye. If the retina becomes detached, you may see floating spots or flashing lights.

You may feel as if a curtain has been pulled over part of what you are looking at. A detached retina can cause loss of sight or blindness if you don't take care of it right away.

Call your eye care professional right away if you are having any vision problems or if you have had a sudden change in your vision.

What can I do about diabetes retina problems?

First, keep your blood glucose and blood pressure as close to normal as you can.

Your eye care professional may suggest laser treatment, which is when a light beam is aimed into the retina of the damaged eye. The beam closes off leaking blood vessels. It may stop blood and fluid from leaking into the vitreous. Laser treatment may slow the loss of sight.

If a lot of blood has leaked into your vitreous and your sight is poor, your eye care professional might suggest you have surgery called a vitrectomy (vih-TREK-tuh-mee). A vitrectomy removes blood and fluids from the vitreous of your eye. Then clean fluid is put back into the eye. The surgery can make your eyesight better.

How do I know if I have retina damage from diabetes?

You may not get any signs of diabetes retina damage or you may get one or more signs:

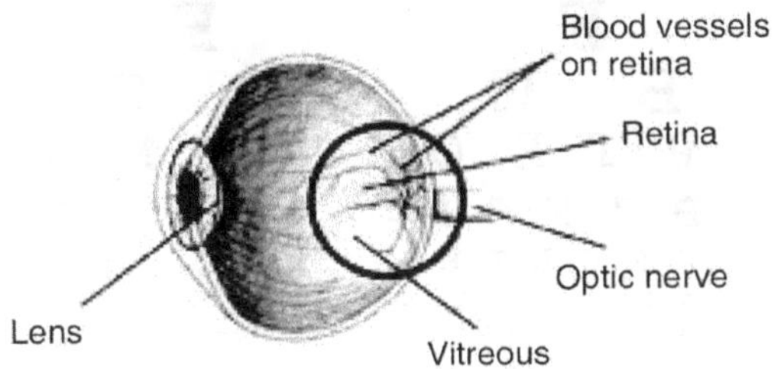

This drawing shows a retina without any damage.

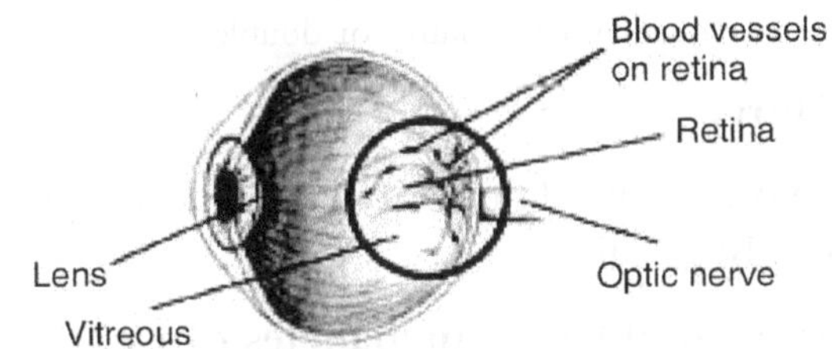

This drawing shows some diabetes damage to a retina.

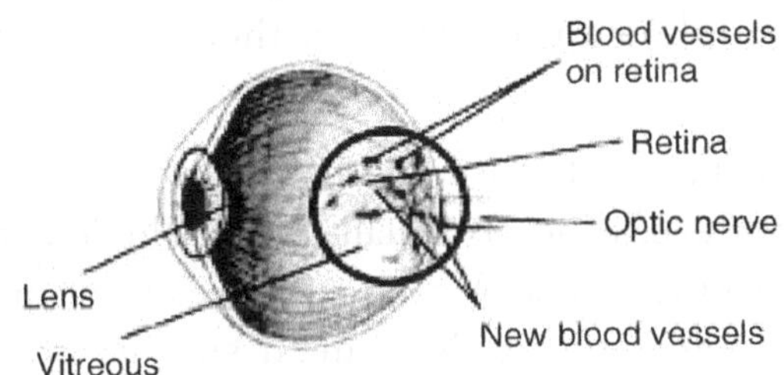

This drawing shows a lot of diabetes damage to a retina.

- blurry or double vision
- rings, flashing lights, or blank spots
- dark or floating spots
- pain or pressure in one or both of your eyes
- trouble seeing things out of the corners of your eyes

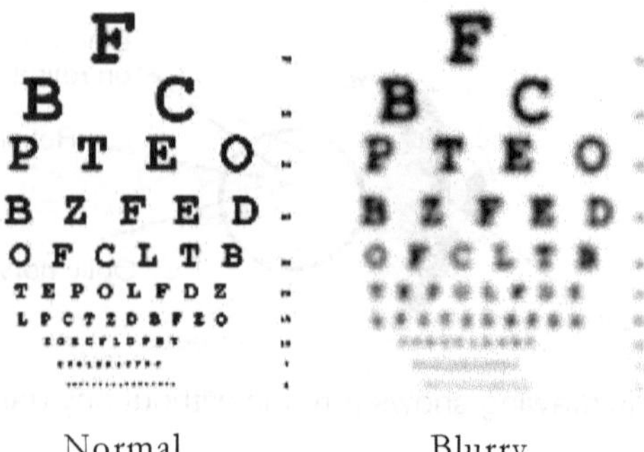

If you have retina damage from diabetes,
you may have blurry or double vision.

Normal Blurry

If you have retina damage from diabetes, you may have blurry or double vision.

What other eye problems can diabetes cause?

You can get two other eye problems-cataracts and glaucoma. People without diabetes can get these eye problems, too. But people with diabetes get them more often and at a younger age.

- A cataract (KAT-uh-rakt) is a cloud over the lens of your eye, which is usually clear. The lens focuses light onto the retina. A cataract makes everything you look at seem cloudy. You need surgery to remove the cataract. During surgery your lens is taken out and a plastic lens, like a contact lens, is put in. The plastic lens stays in your eye all the time. Cataract surgery helps you see clearly again.

Glaucoma (glaw-KOH-muh) starts from pressure building up in the eye. Over time, this pressure damages your eye's main nerve-the optic nerve. The damage first causes you to lose sight from the sides of your eyes. Treating glaucoma is usually simple. Your eye care professional will give you special drops to use every day to lower the pressure in your eye. Or your eye care professional may want you to have laser surgery

(20)

TAKE CARE OF YOUR FEET FOR A LIFETIME

You can take care of your feet!

Do you want to avoid serious foot problems that can lead to a toe, foot, or leg amputation? Take Care of Your Feet for a Lifetime tells you how. It's all about taking good care of your feet.

Foot care is very important for each person with diabetes, but especially if you have:

- Loss of feeling in your feet.
- Changes in the shape of your feet.
- Foot ulcers or sores that do not heal.

Nerve damage can cause you to lose feeling in your feet. You may not feel a pebble inside your sock that is causing a sore. You may not feel a blister caused by poorly fitting shoes. Foot injuries such as these can cause ulcers which may lead to amputation.

Keeping your blood glucose (sugar) in good control and taking care of your feet every day can help you avoid serious foot problems.

Use this guide to make your own plan for taking care of your feet. Helpful tips make it easy! Share your plan with your doctor and health care team and get their help when you need it.

There is a lot you can do to prevent serious problems with your feet. Here's how:

- Take care of your diabetes.
- Check your feet every day.
- Wash your feet every day.
- Keep the skin soft and smooth.
- Smooth corns and calluses gently.
- Trim your toenails each week or when needed.
- Wear shoes and socks at all times.
- Protect your feet from hot and cold.
- Keep the blood flowing to your feet.
- Be more active.
- Be sure to ask your doctor to
- Get started now.
- Tips for Proper Footwear

Ask your doctor about Medicare or other insurance coverage for special footwear.

Take care of your diabetes

- Make healthy lifestyle choices to help keep your blood glucose (sugar), blood pressure, and cholesterol close to normal. Doing so may help prevent or delay diabetes-related foot problems as well as eye and kidney disease.
- Work with your health care team to make a diabetes plan that fits your lifestyle. The team may include your doctor, a diabetes educator, a nurse, a dietitian, a

foot care doctor called a podiatrist (pah-DI-ah-trist), and other specialists. This team will help you to:

- Know when to get checks of your A1C,* blood pressure, and cholesterol.
- Know how and when to test your blood glucose.
- Take your medicines as prescribed.
- Eat regular meals that contain a variety of healthy, low-fat, high-fiber foods including fruits and vegetables each day.
- Get physical activity each day.
- Stop smoking.
- Follow your foot care plan.
- Keep your doctor's visits and have your feet, eyes, and kidneys checked at least once a year.
- Visit your dentist twice a year.
- A1C is a measure of your blood glucose over a 3-month period.

Check your feet every day

- You may have serious foot problems, but feel no pain. Check your feet for cuts, sores, red spots, swelling, and infected toenails. Find a time (evening is best) to check your feet each day. Make checking your feet part of your every day routine.
- If you have trouble bending over to see your feet, use a plastic mirror to help. You also can ask a family member or caregiver to help you.

Check your feet every day.

Make sure to call your doctor right away if a cut, sore, blister, or bruise on your foot does not begin to heal after one day.

Wash your feet every day

- Wash your feet in warm, not hot, water. Do not soak your feet, because your skin will get dry.
- Before bathing or showering, test the water to make sure it is not too hot. You can use a thermometer (90° to 95° F is safe) or your elbow.
- Dry your feet well. Be sure to dry between your toes. Use talcum powder or cornstarch to keep the skin between your toes dry.

Keep the skin soft and smooth

- Rub a thin coat of skin lotion, cream, or petroleum jelly on the tops and bottoms of your feet.
- Do not put lotion or cream between your toes, because this might cause an infection.

Put lotion on the tops and bottoms of your feet.

Smooth corns and calluses gently

- If you have corns and calluses, check with your doctor or foot care specialist about the best way to care for them.
- If your doctor tells you to, use a pumice stone to smooth corns and calluses after bathing or showering. A pumice stone is a type of rock used to smooth the skin. Rub gently, only in one direction, to avoid tearing the skin.
- Do not cut corns and calluses. Don't use razor blades, corn plasters, or liquid corn and callus removers - they can damage your skin.

Gently rub calluses with a pumice stone.

Make sure to call your doctor right away if a cut, sore, blister, or bruise on your foot does not begin to heal after one day.

Trim your toenails each week or when needed

- Trim your toenails with clippers after you wash and dry your feet.
- Trim toenails straight across and smooth them with an emery board or nail file.
- Don't cut into the corners of the toenail.
- If you can't see well, if your toenails are thick or yellowed, or if your nails curve and grow into the skin, have a foot care doctor trim them.
- Trim your toenails straight across and smooth them with a nail file.

Wear shoes and socks at all times

- Wear shoes and socks at all times. Do not walk barefoot - not even indoors - because it is easy to step on something and hurt your feet.
- Always wear socks, stockings, or nylons with your shoes to help avoid blisters and sores.
- Choose clean, lightly padded socks that fit well. Socks that have no seams are best.
- Check the insides of your shoes before you put them on to be sure the lining is smooth and that there are no objects in them.
- Wear shoes that fit well and protect your feet.

Check the inside of your shoes before you put them on.

Protect your feet from hot and cold

- Wear shoes at the beach or on hot pavement.
- Put sunscreen on the top of your feet to prevent sunburn.
- Keep your feet away from radiators and open fires.

- Do not put hot water bottles or heating pads on your feet.
- Wear socks at night if your feet get cold. Lined boots are good in winter to keep your feet warm.
- Check your feet often in cold weather to avoid frostbite.
- Protect your feet when walking on hot surfaces.

Make sure to call your doctor right away if a cut, sore, blister, or bruise on your foot does not begin to heal after one day.

Keep the blood flowing to your feet

- Put your feet up when you are sitting.
- Wiggle your toes for 5 minutes, 2 or 3 times a day. Move your ankles up and down and in and out to improve blood flow in your feet and legs.
- Don't cross your legs for long periods of time.
- Don't wear tight socks, elastic or rubber bands, or garters around your legs.
- Don't smoke. Smoking reduces blood flow to your feet. Ask for help to stop smoking.
- Work with your health care team to control your A1C (blood glucose), blood pressure and cholesterol.
- Put your feet up when you are sitting.

Be more active

- Ask your doctor to help you plan a daily activity program that is right for you.
- Walking, dancing, swimming, and bicycling are good forms of exercise that are easy on the feet.
- Avoid activities that are hard on the feet, such as running and jumping.

- Always include a short warm-up and cool-down period.
- Wear athletic shoes that fit well and that provide good support.
- Walking briskly is a good exercise.

Make sure to call your doctor right away if a cut, sore, blister, or bruise on your foot does not begin to heal after one day.

Be sure to ask your doctor to

- Check the sense of feeling and pulses in your feet at least once a year.
- Tell you if you are likely to have serious foot problems. If you have serious foot problems, your feet should be checked at every visit to your doctor.
- Show you how to care for your feet.
- Refer you to a foot care doctor if needed.
- Decide if special shoes would help your feet stay healthy.

Ask your doctor to check the sense of feeling in your feet.

Get started now

- Begin taking good care of your feet today.
- Set a time every day to check your feet.
- Note the date of your next visit to the doctor.
- Print out the foot care tip sheet and put it on your bathroom or bedroom wall or nightstand as a reminder. Print out and complete the "To Do" list. Get started now.
- Set a date for buying the things you need to take care of your feet: nail clippers, pumice stone, emery board, skin lotion, talcum powder, plastic mirror, socks, athletic shoes, and slippers.
- Most important, stick with your foot care program...

and give yourself a special treat such as a new pair of lightly padded socks with no seams. You deserve it!

Make sure to call your doctor right away if a cut, sore, blister, or bruise on your foot does not begin to heal after one day.

Tips for Proper Footwear

- Proper footwear is very important for preventing serious foot problems. Athletic or walking shoes are good for daily wear. They support your feet and allow them to "breathe."
- Never wear vinyl or plastic shoes, because they don't stretch or "breathe."
- When buying shoes, make sure they are comfortable from the start and have enough room for your toes.
- Don't buy shoes with pointed toes or high heels. They put too much pressure on your toes.

Ask your doctor about Medicare or other insurance coverage for special footwear.

You may need special shoes or shoe inserts to prevent serious foot problems. If you have Medicare Part B insurance, you may be able to get some of the cost of special shoes or inserts paid for. Ask your doctor whether you qualify for

- 1 pair of depth shoes* and 3 pairs of inserts, or
- 1 pair of custom molded shoes (including inserts) and 2 additional pairs of inserts.

If you qualify for Medicare or other insurance coverage, your doctor or podiatrist will tell you how to get your special shoes.

- Depth shoes look like athletic or walking shoes, but have more room in them. The extra room allows for different shaped feet and toes, or for special inserts made to fit your feet.

21

LONG-TERM COMPLICATIONS

Increased life expectancy and longevity have brought with it a number of long-term complications. Some of these are considered to be inevitable consequences of the ageing process. Others in diabetic people are considered long-term complications, as they are specific to the disease. The three most important are eye damage, nerve damage and kidney damage. It is not surprising then that people dread the thought of diabetic complications.

The world has changed, and today the diabetics rightly demand to know all the facts and complications related to the disease. Although medical science has made impressive progress since the discovery of insulin, there is still a long way to go.

Complications may occur with any type of diabetes. The cause of diabetic complications is not completely clear although bad control of diabetes is the most important predisposing factor. Complications are rare in the first few years, and occur more commonly after many years.

At the time the diagnosis is made, the disease of the organ may have been present for a long time, often many years, without the patient having any knowledge of it, and therefore neglected. Hence, it is not surprising that complications can occur in some people even when they are treated with diet alone. For this reason, all doctors and others concerned with treating people with diabetes spend much of their time and effort trying to help them improve their control and keep their blood glucose as near normal as possible.

The best way of detecting complications early is to visit your doctor for regular review. Prevention is clearly better than treatment, and if you can control your diabetes properly you will be less likely to suffer these complications. There are many people on record now who heave gone 50 years or more with insulin-dependent diabetes and are now completely free from any signs of complications.

Regular checks on eyes, blood pressure and feet are a good way of picking up conditions that require treatment at a stage before they have done any serious damage. Just as the control of your diabetes is important, so is the detection and treatment of any complications.

Skin Care

Proper skin care is especially important in preventing bacterial and fungal infections, impaired nerve sensations, dry and itchy skin and other skin problems. Diabetes can cause changes in the tiny blood vessels that supply your skin with nutrients.

Cleanliness of skin is important. When bathing, avoid excessively hot water. Avoid using harsh and highly perfumed soaps. After bathing, gently pat your skin day, particularly in the skin fold in the armpits, the groin, and under the breasts. To stay dry, use talcum powder. Use a lubricating skin oil to moisturise your skin when the humidity is low.

The feet should be washed as it makes the skin soft and more susceptible to infections, particularly in the legs and feet. Your hands too need to be clean. If you have any pressure injuries from shoes or the colour of your skin changes, or you have open wounds, seek professional help. Check your feet frequently, since you may not feel an injury to your feet as readily with diabetic nerve changes that create decreased sensation.

Excessive exposure to the sun can cause burns, which can be serious to a diabetic because of infection, dehydration, and altered diabetic control.

Foot Care

There are major dangers from diabetes, which can affect the feet. The first is due to reduced blood supply from arterial thickening, which leads to poor circulation with cold feet, even in warm weather, and cramps in the calf when walking. The major problem here is arterial sclerosis, and smoking is a more important cause of this than diabetes. In severe cases this can lead to gangrene.

The second way that diabetes can affect the feet is through damage to the nerves, which reduces the feeling of pain and awareness of extremes of temperature. The danger is that any minor damage to the foot, be it from a cut or abrasion or badly fitting shoe, will not cause the usual painful reaction so that damage can result from continued injury or infection spreading. It is essential that you should know whether the sensation in your feet is normal or reduced. Even if there is even a slight numbness of your feet, you should check them daily and seek the advice of someone else to look at the areas that you have difficulty in seeing. If your circulation is poor try hard to keep your feet warm and well protected.

Minor abrasions or cuts can be covered with sterile gauze after using a mild antiseptic cream. Apply cleansing or antiseptic solutions to any openings in the skin, before using the cream.

Avoid using corn plasters as they contain acids which can be dangerous. If you do develop corns and callouses, careful use of pressure-relieving pads help. It is better to get them treated by a chiropodist. They may recommend use of a pumice stone. If they cause persistent pain, redness or swelling, then professional advice from competent specialists is a must.

When your toenails need cutting, always do this after bathing. Keep your toenails trimmed straight across and not too short. Do not cut the corners of your toenails back into the nail grooves as this would injure the soft tissue and allow infection to develop. Avoid using a sharp instrument to clean the free nail edge or the nail grooves.

If your skin is too dry, apply a small amount of emollient cream. For excessive dryness or cracking of the skin on your feet, a moisturing bath oil may also be helpful.

Check and bathe your feet every day. After bathing, dry your feet well, as excessive moisture can set the scene for fungus infections, blisters, and other irritations. Care should be taken to clean between the toes also.

If your skin is moist, dab gently with surgical spirit and then dust lightly with talcum powder.

In cold climates, wear thick woollen socks that are loose fitting, especially if you wear them to bed. If the socks have ridges or seams, wear them inside out. Wear adequate protective outer footwear. Boots or shoes should be warm and waterproof.

Choose shoes which provide good support. They must be broad, long and deep enough. Check that you can wriggle all your toes, and that there is no constriction or excessive rubbing. Check the shoes daily for any small objects, such as tiny stones.

Avoid very hot baths. In winter be careful not to sit too close to the fires or heaters.

Be careful when you walk barefoot on the sands on the

beach, at swimming pools, and in locker rooms. Wear slippers or shoes at all times to prevent foot injuries at home also.

Make sure that your change your socks daily. And avoid wearing socks with holes in them!

Eye Care

The complications specific to diabetes are known as diabetic retinopathy, neuropathy and nephropathy. Retinopathy means damage to the retina at the back of the eye. It is important that you have your eyes checked once a year, for after many years diabetes can affect the retina. The routine eye checks are aimed at picking this up at an early stage before it seriously affects your vision and at a stage where it can be effectively treated.

Retinopathy may occur in people with long-standing diabetes, particularly in those in whom control has not been very good. Abnormalities of the blood flow to the back of the eye develop gradually, and this can lead to deterioration of vision as a result of either disturbance of the function of the eye itself, or of bleeding into the eye from the abnormal blood vessels.

Treatment at this stage with laser usually arrests the process and slows or stops further deterioration.

Some damage to the eyes occurs quite commonly after more than 20 years of diabetes. Retinopathy is, however, usually slight and does not affect vision. Only a very small proportion of people, about 7 per cent, go blind, and these people have had diabetes for 30 years or more.

Vascular changes also can affect the eyes where blood vessels are very tiny and fragile. The fact that diabetes is the leading cause of blindness emphasizes the need for preserving this important faculty.

It is very important for diabetics to have their eyes and vision checked periodically by an ophthalmologist. Be sure that your prescription is up to date, if you wear glasses. If there is a marked blur or change in your vision, consult your physician, for diabetes control changes as well as other conditions can be treated early.

When you have your eyes tested by an ophthalmologist be sure to let him know that you have diabetes. If there are signs of diabetic changes, he may advise a test known as an angiogram where a dye is injected into your arm, and pictures are taken of your eyes to indicate blood vessel changes. Early treatment of these with laser will ensure prevention of progressive eye changes.

If you are handling machinery that may cause flying particles, wear protective eyewear. In bright sunlight always wear sunglasses. Be careful that you do not rub your eyes unnecessarily. Avoid straining your eyes. While reading, writing or working, try to maintain adequate lighting.

If you have shortsightedness it should not make the slightest difference to developing diabetic eye complications. Vision may vary with changes in diabetes control. Severe changes in blood glucose levels can alter the shape of the lens in the eye and thus alter its focusing capacity. It is hence common for those people with high blood glucose levels to have difficulty with distance vision, and this changes completely when their diabetes is controlled and their blood glucose reduced. With this the vision changes again so that a person has difficulty with near vision and therefore with reading. After two or three weeks, vision always returns to the state it was in before diabetes developed.

If you are using contact lenses, the fact that you have diabetes should not interfere with it or influence the sort of lens you are given. What should be of more importance are the local factors affecting your eyes and vision. A qualified optician or an ophthalmologist can guide you in these matters.

Although glaucoma can occur commonly in people who do not have diabetes, there is a slightly increased risk in those who do. This generally affects those who have advanced diabetic eye problems.

Sometimes the eye drops that are administered in your eyes to dilate the pupil for a proper view of the retina can precipitate an attack of glaucoma. If there is pain in the affected eye along with blurring of vision coming on some hours after the drops have been put in, seek urgent medical advice, as it is reversible with rapid treatment, but can cause serious damage if not treated immediately.

Dental Care

Your teeth and mouth tissues must be in good health to prevent dental problems that could have serious complications, such as gingivitis, which is inflammation of the gums that begins around the teeth and causes bleeding. This can also lead to tooth decay and complications. A blessing in disguise for diabetics is that since they avoid sweets, they have less chance of dental caries.

When you visit your dentist, be sure to tell him that you have diabetes before any dental procedures are done. Though diabetes will not affect your dental treatment, it is important to remove all possibility of a hypo while in the dentist's chair. If you are on insulin, warn him that you cannot run over a snack or meal time. If your treatment needs a general anaesthetic, this is usually done in a hospital as you are on insulin.

See your dentist at least twice a year. Get your teeth and gums checked up, and have teeth cleaned at least twice a year. If you find any scratches, sores or other injuries appearing in your mouth, seek professional advice.

Brush your teeth regularly, at least twice a day, following instructions of your dentist. Carry a toothbrush with you, so that you can brush during your workday or when away from home, after meals. Floss your teeth daily, and avoid using too-hard toothbrushes that might irritate delicate oral tissues.

Kidney Complications

Diabetics have more kidney diseases than non-diabetics. This occurs because blood vessels serving the kidneys often are affected, and recurrent infections of the urinary tract can be more common. Diabetic nephropathy can cause severe damage to the kidneys, which in the first instance makes them more leaky so that albumin appears in the urine. At a later stage it may affect the function of the kidneys, and in severe cases lead to kidney failure.

There are several ways in which diabetes may affect the kidneys, and they will show up in the routine urine and blood tests.

You are at risk of infection when a lot of glucose in your urine spreads from the bladder up to the kidneys, leading to cystitis (infection and inflammation of the urinary bladder) and pyelonephritis (inflammation of the central part of the kidneys). Sometimes chronic kidney infections produce very little in the way of symptoms, and can only be revealed by routine tests.

High blood glucose in people with poorly controlled and long-standing diabetes can affect the small blood vessels supplying the kidneys. This may not produce any symptoms but will be discovered in a routine urine test.

A special test detects the presence of microalbuminuria, which is a microscopic amount of albumin (protein) in the urine. This test is useful as it can detect the very early signs of kidney damage.

When the kidney disease is severe or acute, massive amounts of albumin may be lost in the urine, which may make the urine froth and lead to accumulation of fluid in the body and oedema (swelling due to fluid retention) around the ankles.

With kidney failure, a diabetic may have to go in for dialysis or eventual transplantation both of which are suitable forms of treatment.

The insulin requirement often diminishes when the kidney function is compromised. Orals drugs like chlorpropamide, which are excreted by the kidneys, and biguanides, are best avoided when the kidney function is impaired. The short acting Glipizide is preferred. One should also control one's high blood pressure.

Complications Related to Nerves

Damage to the neural pathways is known as neuropathy. Diabetic neuropathy, by leading to loss of feeling, particularly in the feet, makes affected people very susceptible to infections, and rarely gangrene with the subsequent need for an amputation. It can also cause impotence.

Neuropathy can affect nerves supplying any part of the body, but is generally referred to as either peripheral or 'autonomic'.

Peripheral neuropathy affect nerves supplying muscles and skin. Diabetes may affect the nerves of the limbs, especially the lower ones. This gives rise to tingling and numbness of the feet, what is also termed as 'pins and needles', usually worse at night. There is weakness of the legs and unsteadiness, due to the numbing of sensations. This numbness and loss of pain may lead to disorganisation of the small joints of the foot. The feet and ankle may be swollen, yet the pain is absent or minimal. In such a situation, injuries to the foot or sole may go unnoticed.

Some diabetics may find climbing the stairs an ordeal due to a sharp pain and weakness of the thighs. Sometimes only one leg causes problems when a single nerve in it gets affected.

A warm, not hot, bath followed by a massage with oil or lanolin helps to keep the skin of the feet supple. Drugs can relieve the pain in the limbs, which are typically worse at night.

Autonomic neuropathy affects nerves supplying organs such as the bladder, the bowel and the heart. The autonomic nervous system regulates the unconscious functions of the body, such as breathing the beating of the heart, the rate of glandular activity, and the contraction and dilation of the blood vessels.

The best way of detecting complications early is to visit your doctor or clinic for regular review. Strict control of your diabetes is equally important for the prevention and treatment of this complication and treatment of this complication. Remember, it can be made worse by moderate or high consumption of alcohol.

Bowel neuropathy is one of the features of autonomic neuropathy. This may occur in some people with long-standing diabetes, where there is loss of function of the nerves that regulate the activity of your bowels. The symptoms are indigestion, occasionally vomiting, and occurrences of alternating constipation and diarrhoea. Sometimes, before diarrhoea sets in, there are rumblings and gurgling in the stomach, and commonly this responds quite well to a short course of antibiotics. A high-fibre diet is encouraged to prevent constipation.

Diabetes ranks high as a cause of impotence. Temporary impotence, another result of nerve damage, can occur when diabetes is in poor control, and is due to general weakness. Due to anxiety also impotence may result. In long-standing diabetics impotence may be due to the involvement of autonomic nervous system or of the blood vessels. Many drugs administered for high blood pressure, allergy or psychological problems or even tobacco can contribute to the problem.

Heart and Arterial Complications

In many people with diabetes complications occur in blood

vessels. Since diabetics are more prone to problems with blood vessels, such conditions appear earlier, and advance more rapidly than in non-diabetics. And since both the large and small blood vessels can be involved, complications, such as hypertension and atherosclerosis, often are the principal problems in the care of the diabetics.

Vascular disease (disease of the blood vessels) causes other complications of the circulatory system, including heart attack. Women with diabetes rather than those without it have more heart disease, especially after menopause. Also, as there are changes in the arteries due to diabetes, some diabetics have peripheral circulatory problems, especially in their legs.

Narrowing or hardening of the arteries is a normal part of growing older, and this process, leading to poor circulation in the feet and legs, can affect the arteries to the feet. Similarly, also to other parts of the body. The causes of arterial disease are not very well known, but it is true that smoking and poor diabetes control make it worse. So stop smoking, control your blood glucose, and keep active.

Occlusion or blockage of more than one artery and multiple blocks are common in diabetic premenopausal women. Besides, these large blood vessels may be affected in long-standing diabetes. The heart muscle can also get affected; white the nerves, which control the heart function, may get damaged.

Decreased blood supply to the heart may give rise to breathlessness or discomfort or heaviness in the chest, or arms, or jaws, or shoulders, on walking or negotiating stains. When you rest, these symptoms disappear. If the blood supply to the heart is drastically reduced then a part of the heart muscle may be destroyed. This infarction (death of tissues) of the heart muscles gives rise to a severe and prolonged chest pain even while resting. Other complications could be sweating breathlessness, vomiting, fainting or sudden death. The pain may be minimal or absent in diabetics.

Some drugs administered for heart problems may suppress the warning signals of hypoglycaemia. Hence, it is important for a diabetic to report to his doctor when he has chest pain or discomfort at rest.

Care of the Elderly

Elderly diabetics require special attention, as many of them have chronic ill health. Past the age of 60, there is continued increase in the incidence of diabetes. It is three times as frequent as in middle age.

Generally though, there is a decline in the severity of the disease. It is relatively mild in regard to urinary sugar, fewer cases require insulin, and more can be managed on dietary control. Chances are less of ketosis, and there are lesser incidents of insulin shock.

Though the disease itself poses fewer difficulties, the ageing process creates a new set of problems in relation to the disease. The possibility of shock may be remote but the consequences may be far more severe. With age, arteries become more brittle, and shock may cause serious organic damage as a result – either a heart attack or a stroke.

In an elderly diabetic, the stress of an acute illness, an accident or an operation may cause a change in this diabetes, necessitating an increase of insulin or some other compensation in treatment. The complications arising from arteriosclerosis are more frequent and more severe than for the non-diabetic. Injury and infection, which caused very little problems for the younger diabetics, now are hazardous because of the decrease in blood circulation. The feet are especially vulnerable as circulation here is usually most sluggish.

There are many ways that an elderly diabetic can adopt to protect himself from these complications. By keeping his weight normal or a little below is, he can help his circulatory system.

He should guard against injuries and infections, especially of the feet. He should wear comfortable-fitting shoes, avoid socks that are tight, too large or wrinkled, wear slippers or shoes always, take care will cutting toenails, avoid extremes of cold and heat, change socks daily, and be careful in choosing his work or recreation that will not cause injury, especially to the feet. An important fact that he should remember is that if he has any injury or infection, then its treatment should be left strictly to the physician. A close contact with the doctor or physician is particularly important for the elderly patient.

The elderly are less active than the young, and so they need less kcals. After 40 years of age, the kcal requirement of a person falls by 5 per cent, after 50 by 10 per cent, after 60 by 15 per cent.

Many elderly people living alone often like beverages and bread, and avoid cooking a regular meal. Many of them are constipated, and they need to consume more liquids and fibre-rich foods to stimulate bowel movement. It is advisable to have liquid during the early part of the day to prevent frequent visits to the toilet at night.

22

RESEARCH AND NEW ADVANCEMENTS

A diabetic owes his well-being and existence to ongoing research in diabetes. Those involved in it include the International Diabetes Federation, Belgium, the National Research Councils, universities and the pharmaceutical industry. Due to current research efforts, prospects for not only treating diabetes but also preventing it look promising. Researchers are interested in studying the various aspects of the diabetes, which is a complex disease. Their students range from the genetic details in unborn children to improved drug therapies for those who have had diabetes for many years.

Diabetes is not a new disease but current knowledge about it and its treatment has evolved over several centuries. In the past 100 years research has led to better ways of treating diabetes. In 1869, a German pathologist, Paul Langerhans, made the most significant research when he discovered that some cells, known as beta cells, in the pancreas were different from other cells, and that they produced insulin in our bodies. Then two Canadian physicians, Sir Frederick Grant Banting and Charles Herbert Best, extracted insulin from the pancreas of animals and injected it into dogs. They found that the insulin reduced the amount of sugar in the dog's blood. Since then, man has progressed a long way in his research. Today, this insulin is what saves the lives of thousands of diabetics all around the world.

from other cells, and that they produced insulin in our bodies. Then two Canadian physicians, Sir Frederick Grant Banting and Charles Herbert Best, extracted insulin from the pancreas of animals and injected it into dogs. They found that the insulin reduced the amount of sugar in the dog's blood. Since then, man has progressed a long way in his research. Today, this insulin is what saves the lives of thousands of diabetics all around the world.

Today, although we have not yet mastered diabetes, we have learned to control it. It is no longer almost invariably fatal. We can detect it, treat it, lessen its symptoms and control them, reduce its complications, and cope with most of its problems. What is more, this can be done with a minimum of intrusion into the ordinary routines of daily living. Today's diabetic can now live a longer, fuller and more nearly normal life than was ever before imagined possible.

Weight normalisation and adequate diet are the main goals in controlling diabetes. Researchers in nutrition are studying the effects of various aspects of diet on the way diabetics utilise the foods they eat. While some suggest low carbohydrate diets, some others suggest lowering the ratio of saturated to unsaturated fatty acids. Plans are under way to try them, and eventually these trials may bring better ways of controlling the disease.

There are some scientists of the opinion that a deficiency of fibre in the diet may affect insulin availability. They also feel that increased fibre content in the diet may improve blood glucose control in those who have diabetes. Certain data indicate that the addition of certain components of fibre improves control of glucose, and reduces the need for insulin and oral anti-diabetic agents.

Research is going on to seek better ways to prevent serious birth defects and postnatal problems that sometimes occur in infants of diabetic mothers. There are steps being taken to improve home blood-testing devices and insulin delivery programmes, so that expected mothers can maintain better control of their blood sugar. With better management and techniques for administering insulin, more diabetic mothers will be ale to carry their pregnancies more normally, and fewer Caesarean sections need be necessary among them. Researchers are evolving better methods to monitor foetal health so that pregnancies among diabetics may be subjected to decreased risk.

Research Focus on Causes and Cure

Research is an ongoing process, and this applies to diabetes also. Basic researches are continuing to seek and gather information on causes, and to find better ways of controlling diabetes. They are studying at the mechanisms of insulin secretion, insulin action and resistance, and glucose balance. They are looking into how insulin receptor sites are altered by drugs.

Researchers believe that certain individual have an increased risk of developing diabetes. They are studying the susceptibility factors so that those at risk of developing diabetes can be identified, and appropriate preventive steps can be taken. Now there is considerable focus on certain viruses, reactions of the immune system, and environmental factors, which could be possible contributors and causes in the development of diabetes. Vaccines are being developed and tested, and there is hope of developing an immunisation against the viruses that produce juvenile-onset diabetes.

Some research work has been done of extending the honeymoon period, using anti-viral agents and drugs that interfere with the body's immune responses. The results, though showing no positive benefit, do suggest that the immuno-suppressive therapy may prolong the honeymoon period in some patients.

A lot of research is going on in seeking ways to cure diabetes completely. It is an exciting period in diabetic research, and we may continue to look forward to improvements in our understanding of the disease, which does not mean that at a later date a solution to this will not be found. Research is being done towards this achievement. The diabetic cures that have occurred are more in the nature of remissions. Permanent remissions do happen, although they are rare. For instance, a diabetic person, who had an adrenal tumour and was operated upon, was cured of his diabetes. There is an explanation for this. There are now forms of adrenal tumour, where the tumour produces adrenaline and noradrenaline, both of which inhibit insulin secretion by the pancreas. The other adrenal tumour produces a form of diabetes, which is reversible on removal of the tumour.

There are a number of other rare conditions often associated with disturbances of other hormone-producing glands in the body. In these cases diabetes can be cured after appropriate therapy of the hormonal disturbances. For instances, it is generally believed that the stress of pregnancy may provoke latent diabetes. Remissions also take place in juvenile diabetes after insulin treatment is begun. But the disease invariably returns.

In several cases of mild diabetes, the simple dietary measures of avoiding concentrated sugars and reducing calories are sufficient to eliminate abnormal blood sugar and other symptoms permanently or for many years. In other apparently similar cases, the ailment may suddenly flare up in severity. Even in some cases of flagrant diabetes, single dietary measures may bring a total disappearance of the disease, which is maintained as the years go by.

Sometimes, illness, pregnancy or stress, emotional as well

as physical, may provoke the symptoms of diabetes for a brief period after which they vanish only to reappear again at some future date.

There are some who believe that certain cases of insulin-dependent diabetes may be caused by a combination of genetic predisposition, viruses and auto-immune response where the body attacks its own cells as foreign objects. Researchers are studying viruses suspected of damaging the insulin-producing cells of the pancreas. They are also studying those viruses that cause mumps and measles, which, they feel, might also contribute to the onset of diabetes. They are studying the relationship between viruses and auto-immunity to find out if there is an important interaction between them. However, the immune system being complex, the diabetes develops in different ways in different people so that many fields of research will continue.

If a virus were isolated which caused diabetes, then it should be possible to produce a vaccine, which could be given to children to prevent them from developing diabetes later on in life.

Pancreas Transplant

Pancreatic transplantation is still in the experimental stages. The pancreas is very delicate, and as the seat of many digestive juices, it has a tendency to digest itself if damaged even a little. The narrow duct through which these juices pass has to be joined to the intestines in a very intricate way so that the enzymes do not ooze out. Provided everything goes well, the body will still react against transplant, and hence many immuno-suppressants have to be given. Some of these, particularly steroids, given in high doses, tend to cause diabetes or make existing ones worse. In many cases, where the transplantation of pancreas has taken place, the grafts do quite well, and most people discontinue insulin injections, and resume a normal diet, at least for a while. Yet there are a number of problems attached to this form of treatment. Treatment to prevent rejection of the graft is long-term, expensive, and currently limited to experimental study.

Islet Transplant

The islets of Langerhans are a cluster of cells scattered through the tissues of pancreas, and they produce the hormone insulin. Many cases of diabetes mellitus are caused when these cells fail to produce enough insulin to help the body burn up starches and sugar, and convert them into energy.

Since it is the islets of Langerhans in the pancreas rather than the whole pancreas that produce insulin, it would be logical to transplant the islets rather than the whole pancreas in a diabetic. By enclosing the islets in a porous membrane and transplanting them into an animal with diabetes, it is possible to show that the insulin can get out of the bag of islets, and normalise the blood glucose at the same time, as nutrients from the bloodstream can get in to sustain the islets. While this is going on the membrane keeps at bay the cells responsible for tissue rejection. Unfortunately, after a while the membrane tends to get clogged with scar tissue, and the islet graft stops working. Until there has been a major breakthrough in the transplantation of tissues from one individual to another, the hazards of long-term immuno-suppressive therapy for someone receiving either a pancreas transplant or on islet transplant are far greater those of having diabetes treated with insulin.

Artificial Pancreas

There is a great deal of research going on amongst several bio-engineering groups to develop a system with an artificial pancreas to maintain blood glucose levels in which administered insulin is controlled by the prevailing glucose level. Units in which blood is taken continuously have been developed, and its glucose content determined by a computerised device. Another computer then calculates the requirement of insulin, and injects with a pump the appropriate amount of insulin.

These systems are expensive and suitable only for short-term studies. Currently, they have little value to the average person with diabetes. Researchers, based on their knowledge of such equipment, are hoping to develop smaller systems that can be implanted, to measure glucose and automatically administer insulin. At present available machines are rather crude, heavy and bulky, very complex, and extremely expensive. The major value is for research purposes since they are quite unsuitable at present as devices for long-term control.

Insulin Pumps

Insulin pumps have been transplanted into people as part of research studies, and there has been some encouraging progress in this field. These are still in the experimental stage, and the devices are constantly being improved.

At present, there are three portable insulin pumps available. They are open, closed, and combination pumps. Some diabetologists are of the opinion that a completely closed system that includes a glucose sensor to reflect the constant blood sugar level would be ideal. This would be connected to a computer that would move insulin out of a reservour into the circulatory system on demand. Such a unit could well control diabetes. The greatest hurdle in developing this system has been devising a dependable sensor. Open or semi-closed systems having pumps that can be programmed or adjusted by the patient to release doses of insulin based on self-monitored glucose levels have also been developed.

The current insulin implantable pumps require the patient to monitor capillary blood glucose and adjust the rate of insulin infusion. Instead of constantly testing blood glucose, continuous blood glucose sensor is being considered. Their sensors could be used with an external or an implantable insulin infusion pump. Some pumps utilise refillable insulin reservoirs and techniques for adjusting dosage. Most of these insulin pumps are small and handy, about the size of a package of cigarettes.

These pumps are useful as a continuous infusion of insulin throughout the day and an extra dose at meal time can be programmed. They allow the body to use its sugar more normally at all times; and permit constant night-time dosage. The risks of developing complications from diabetes are therefore minimised.

Pumps usually require having a needle implanted in the patient's skin. This must be changed or removed often for activities, or every two-three days to avoid damage or infection. The negative factor is that the person using the pump must change the needle position every day or every several days. Care should be taken to see that the needle does not get dislodged, and they must set dials appropriately before meals and at other times. Although promising, the major disadvantages are cost and complexity.

Researchers are trying to develop a small electronic device which can be implanted under the skin and which can continuously monitor the level of glucose in the blood. Not only arc there technical problems in achieving an accurate reflection of blood glucose level by such a subcutaneous-implanted glucose sensor, but also the further problem of connecting it to a supply of insulin to be released according to the demand is formidable. Let us not give up hopes though!

New and Oral Insulins

Improved varieties of insulin are undergoing evaluation. There are short-acting or long-acting varieties or specific insulin-like molecules, designed with specific aims in consideration. One such insulin analogue has recently been introduced in India. Soon the widespread use of insulin analogues could become a reality for correcting hyperglycaemia without the risk of hypoglycaemia.

For some years now purer insulins are being developed with patterns of absorption varying from the very quick-acting to the very long-acting formulations. Biosynthetic human insulins have replaced the animal insulins for most patients. These are manufactured by pharmaceuticals by interfering with the genetic codes of bacteria and yeasts and inserting material that instructs the organisms to produce insulin. By inserting the genetic material coding for human insulin scientists can get the organisms to produce more human insulin, as well as new insulin. Produced in large quantities these will become less expensive, and its use will become more widespread.

The benefits from this remarkable advance in scientific manufacturing are already clear. Trials show that one of these insulins is absorbed much more quickly than any of the fast-acting insulin, is very good for covering meals, and can be given immediately before the meal rather than 15-30 minutes before.

Some claim that it is possible to get away from insulin injections either by using nasal insulin sprays or by producing some form of insulin, which is active when taken orally. There is no doubt that a small proportion of any insulin put in the nose is absorbed through the membranes into the bloodstream and can lower the blood glucose. Unfortunately, only a little of what is put in the nose is absorbed, and is therefore not an efficient and good way of administering insulin. Since the absorption is erratic, the blood glucose is not very stable. Experiments with insulin suppositories show that they too can lower the blood glucose without the need for injections, but again the absorption is not total and the response is erratic. It is possible that better methods will be found for increasing the absorption from these sites, and making this a possible alternative mode of insulin administration.

Regarding oral insulin, it is possible to prevent the stomach digesting the insulin by incorporating it into a fat or lipid droplet which enables it to be absorbed from the gut without being broken down by the digestive juices. Again, here too, the absorption is erratic, the whole lipid droplet with the insulin is absorbed, and there nothing to tell when the insulin will be released from the droplet and become active. At present it seems unlikely that effective oral insulin will be developed in the foreseeable future.

Technological Advances

All the modern insulin pumps rely heavily on microchips to control the rate of infusion. There are microcomputer programmes, which help to store and analyse home blood monitoring records. Soon it would be possible to stimulate the blood glucose responses to different insulin injections, and in this way make way for exploring the effect of different types and doses of insulin, and stimulating the body's responses.

Microcomputers are being used to help record and analyse information from the diabetes clinic as well as to plan and manage monitoring of diabetes care, and to write letters. Experiments are being carried out in the use of so-called 'expert systems' to transfer the expert knowledge and reasoning of specialists to general practitioners to facilitate their management of people with diabetes within general practice, without the need for them to visit hospital diabetes clinics, so often.

The technologists introduced the mass spectrometer in clinics several years ago, and this has benefited the diabetic masses. It is a very complicated machine that is used to measure minute amounts of very similar substances present in the bloodstream or in other body parts. It is often used in measuring amounts of naturally occurring isotopes that can be given to diabetics to find out their body's metabolism in great detail. Earlier, this type of study could only be carried out by injecting radioactive isotopes, which could then be monitored in the body, as they were metabolised. These radioisotopes can have harmful effects on cells in the body. Even the smallest amount

23

PREVENT DIABETES PROBLEMS: KEEP YOURSELF HEALTHY

What should I do each day to stay healthy with diabetes?

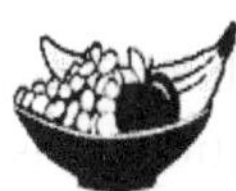

Follow the healthy eating plan that you and your doctor or dietitian have workd out

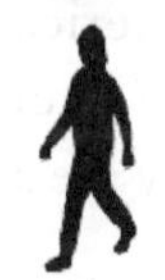

Be active a total of 30 minutes most days. Ask your doctor what activities are best for you.

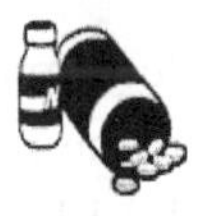

Take your medicines as directed

Check your blood glucose every day. Each time you check your blood glucose, write the number in your record book.

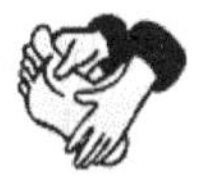

Check your feet every day for cuts, blisters, sores, swelling redness, or sore to enails.

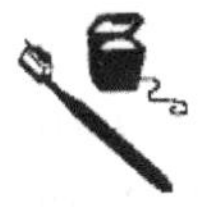

Brush and floss your teeth every day

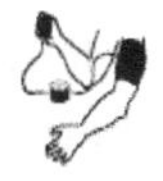

Control you blood pressure and cholesterol

Don't smoke.

24

HOW TO TELL IF YOU HAVE PRE-DIABETES

While diabetes and pre-diabetes occur in people of all ages and races, some groups have a higher risk for developing the disease than others. Diabetes is more common in African Americans, Latinos, Native Americans, and Asian Americans/Pacific Islanders, as well as the aged population. This means they are also at increased risk for developing pre-diabetes.

There are two different tests your doctor can use to determine whether you have pre-diabetes: the fasting plasma glucose test (FPG) or the oral glucose tolerance test (OGTT). The blood glucose levels measured after these tests determine whether you have a normal metabolism, or whether you have pre-diabetes or diabetes. If your blood glucose level is abnormal following the FPG, you have impaired fasting glucose (IFG); if your blood glucose level is abnormal following the OGTT, you have impaired glucose tolerance (IGT).

Pre-diabetes is a serious medical condition that can be treated. The good news is that the recently completed Diabetes Prevention Program study conclusively showed that people with pre-diabetes can prevent the development of type 2 diabetes by making changes in their diet and increasing their level of physical activity. They may even be able to return their blood glucose levels to the normal range.

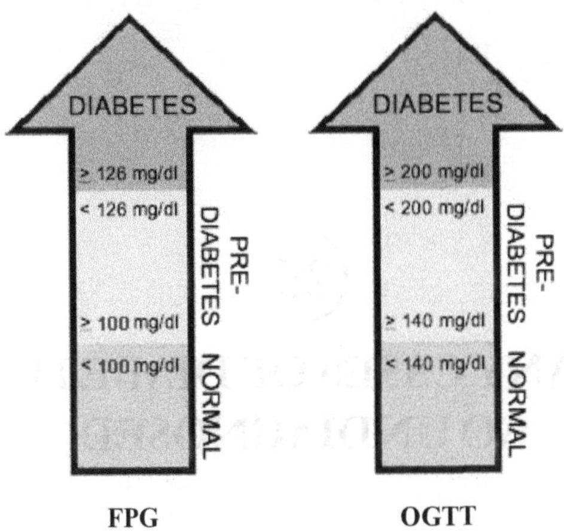

FPG **OGTT**

While the DPP also showed that some medications may delay the development of diabetes, diet and exercise worked better. Just 30 minutes a day of moderate physical activity, coupled with a 5-10% reduction in body weight, produced a 58% reduction in diabetes.

25

MANY CASES OF DIABETES GO UNDIAGNOSED

A report by the Institute of Health and Welfare has found the number of diagnosed cases of diabetes in Australia has more than doubled since 1990.

The disease is now causing or contributing to one in 11 deaths in Australia, with 700,000 reported cases of diabetes in the country.

Doctors are not surprised by the report, but the president of the Australian Medical Association (AMA), Rosanna Capolingua, says it is a wake-up call.

"For those people who have got diabetes now I guess it's, 'let's get you healthier, let's get you fitter, let's get you to lose weight. Your diabetes will be much better managed. In fact, in some cases, you may even find that it ebbs away if we get on to you now'," she said.

"And for the rest of Australia that aren't yet diagnosed but are part of our obesity and overweight problem and our lifestyle problem, the message is - wake up Australia."

Not surprisingly, the spike has been driven by an increase in Type 2 diabetes, a form of the disease that is largely preventable.

But experts believe for every confirmed case, there is an undiagnosed one.

Researcher Lynelle Moon says some parts of the population are more susceptible to the disease than others.

"Type 2 diabetes is largely preventable. The main risk factors are overweight and obesity and physical inactivity," she says.

"The standout group is Aboriginal and Torres Strait Islander peoples who have diabetes prevalence rates that are three times that of other Australians.

"They also have higher death and hospitalisation rates around 11 to 12 times higher."

The 2008 report also found poorer Australians are twice as likely to develop diabetes than the well-off.

Ms Moon says there were some shocking results in remote communities.

"The difference between diabetes rates between people living in the city and more remote areas was not terrifically different," she said.

"What was different was hospitalisation rates which were two to three times as high in remote areas as in the metropolitan areas, and the difference in death rates was being around two to four times higher."

Diabetes can lead to heart disease, kidney failure, blindness, amputations, oral health problems and impotence.

In 2004-2005, diabetes and complications accounted for one in 11 deaths and 500,000 hospital admissions.

"The costs just to our health care system was $907 million in that one year," Ms Moon said.

26

FREQUENTLY ASKED QUESTIONS ABOUT NUTRITION

Why do I need to see a dietitian?

Registered dietitians (RDs) have training and expertise in how the body uses food. RDs who understand diabetes can teach you how the food you eat changes your blood glucose level and how to coordinate your diabetes medications and eating. Do you know how many calories you should eat each day? How to cut down on the fat in your meals? How to make eating time more interesting? An RD can help you learn the answers to these, and lots of other questions. Your dietitian will work with you to create a healthy eating plan that includes your favorite foods.

Can I eat foods with sugar in them?

For almost every person with diabetes, the answer is yes! Eating a piece of cake made with sugar will raise your blood glucose level. So will eating corn on the cob, a tomato sandwich, or lima beans. The truth is that sugar has gotten a bad reputation. People with diabetes can and do eat sugar. In your body, it becomes glucose, but so do the other foods mentioned above. With sugary foods, the rule is moderation. Eat too much, and 1) you'll send your blood glucose level up higher than you expected; 2) you'll fill up but without the nutrients that come with vegetables and grains; and 3) you'll gain weight. So, don't pass up a slice of birthday cake. Instead, eat a little less bread or potato, and replace it with the cake. Taking a brisk walk to burn some calories is also always helpful.

Why does losing weight help my diabetes?

Weight loss helps people with diabetes in two important ways. First, it lowers insulin resistance. This allows your natural insulin (in people with type 2 diabetes) to do a better job lowering blood glucose levels. If you take a diabetes medicine, losing weight lowers blood glucose and may allow you to reduce the amount you're taking, or quit taking it altogether. Second, it improves blood fat and blood pressure levels. People with diabetes are about twice as likely to get cardiovascular disease as most people. Lowering blood fats and blood pressure is a way to reduce that risk.

How can I cut the fat in my diet?

Here are some beginning hints. See a dietitian for more advice. Stir-fry foods in tiny amounts of oil and lots of seasonings. Choose nonfat or low-fat selections, such as nonfat or 1% milk or low-fat cheese. Keep portion sizes on target. Avoid fried foods -- bake, grill, broil, or roast vegetables and meat instead.

Are some fats better than others?

Yes. Unsaturated fats are the healthiest for your body. This includes both monounsaturated and polyunsaturated fats. You can find these "healthy fats" in foods like nuts, vegetable oils, olives and avocados.

The fats to cut back on are the saturated and trans fats. Saturated fats are found in full-fat dairy products like ice cream, half and half, sour cream, cheese, and meats, chicken skin, bacon and lard. Trans fats are found in margarines and shortening as well as many processed packaged foods and sweets. Trying to cut back on how much saturated and trans fat you eat is important to help reduce your risk of heart attack and stroke.

What foods can I eat a lot of?

Forget about eating with abandon. The key to healthy living is moderation. Air-popped popcorn may be low in fat, but it still has calories. And calories count. If you can control the portion sizes of the food you eat, you will be able to eat a wider variety of foods, including your favorites, and still keep your blood sugar in your target range.

What can I do if I overeat over the holidays?

Put on your walking shoes and head for the pavement. Being more active helps lower your blood sugar, blood pressure and cholesterol. Physical activity uses up extra sugar in your blood and helps your insulin work better.

Can I use low calorie sweeteners?

Low calorie sweeteners are safe for everyone except people with phenylketonuria, who should not use aspartame. Calorie-free sweeteners like aspartame, saccharin, sucralose and acesulfame-K won't increase your blood glucose level. The sugar alcohols—xylitol, mannitol, and sorbitol—have some calories and do slightly increase your blood glucose level. Eating too much of any of these can cause gas and diarrhea.

How much weight should I lose each week?

Limiting your weight loss to 1/2 to 1 pound a week will keep you healthy, and let you enjoy the foods you love in small amounts. A slow steady weight loss is the key to keeping lost weight off.

Can I drink alcohol?

Yes, in moderation. Moderation is defined as two drinks a day for men and one drink a day for women. A drink is a 5-ounce glass of wine, a 12-ounce light beer, or 1-1/2 ounces of 80-proof distilled spirits. Make sure that your medications don't require avoiding alcohol, and get your doctor's okay.

Isn't glucose control easier if I eat the same things every day?

Probably, but this method of blood glucose control isn't very nutritious, not to mention boring. One of the keys to nutrition is eating a variety of foods each day. By checking your blood glucose two hours after starting to eat a meal, you can learn how different foods affect you. Over time, you will be able to predict how foods, and combinations of foods, affect your blood glucose level.

What vitamins will help my diabetes?

If you have a vitamin or mineral deficiency, it could be causing problems with your glucose control. For instance, one study found that taking the trace element chromium improved glucose control in subjects who had a chromium deficiency. More studies need to be done. If you choose a variety of fruits, vegetables, grains, and meat each day, and keep your blood sugar close to your target range, you probably don't need to take vitamin supplements because of diabetes.

Are there herbs that will help my diabetes?

Many herbs supposedly have glucose-lowering effects, but there arc not enough data on any herb to recommend it for use in people with diabetes. Herbs are not considered food by the Food and Drug Administration and are not tested for quality or content. Therefore, products can be promoted as helping health conditions without having to show evidence of this. Discuss the herbal dietary supplements with your doctor or dietitian before trying them. They may interact poorly with your diabetes medication.

GLOSSARY

Acetone : a substance formed in the body during wasting or after excessive vomiting. It is one of the chemicals called ketones formed when the body uses up fat for energy. It smells like nail-varnish remover, is passed in the urine, and can sometimes be detected on the patient's breath.

Acidosis : a condition in which the blood is more acid than normal, owing to an excess of carbon dioxide produced in the body. This disturbance of the body's normal acid/alkali balance is serious.

Adrenaline : a hormone that is produced by the adrenal glands. When the body is under the kind of stress produced by shock, anger or fear, the glands increase their secretion of adrenaline and pass it into the blood, which carries it to every part of the body. The hormone rapidly prepares the body for emergency action, such as flight or fight, by speeding up the beating of the heart.

Albumin : a protein that is present in many plant and animal tissues. It occurs in the blood as serum albumin, in which form it helps to regulate the distribution of water in the body.

Alpha cell : the cell that produces glucagons, found in the islets of Langerhans in the pancreas.

Amino acid : any of about 20 complex chemical substances that form the building blocks of proteins, compounds essential for keeping the body running. When food is digested, the protein in it is broken down into amino acids, which are then reassembled in different combinations to make the particular kinds of protein required by human muscles, red blood cells, and other body tissues.

Antigens : a substance that stimulates the production of antibodies when it enters the body. When antigens like viruses, bacteria, dust, fungi, etc., appear in the body, the antibodies produced, or already present, move into action and neutralise them. This protective mechanism is the basis of immunity to infectious diseases.

Arteriosclerosis : the medical name for the condition commonly called hardening of the arteries. In the later years of life, the arteries become narrow and less flexible and are therefore not so efficient at their job of piping oxygen-rich blood through the body. Minerals and fatty deposits build up in the arteries, making them narrower and their walls thicker and less resilient.

Artery : any blood vessel that carries oxygen-rich blood away from the heart to the rest of body.

Aspartame : a low-calorie intense sweetener.

Atherosclerosis : a condition in which deposits of fatty substances form inside an artery and obstruct the flow of blood.

Autonomic neuropathy : damage to the system of nerves which regulate many autonomic functions of the body such as stomach emptying, sexual function (potency) and blood pressure control.

Bacteria : microscopic organisms commonly called microbes, or, if they cause infection or disease, germs.

Beta cells : located in the pancreas and responsible for the production of the supply of insulin for the body.

Biguanides : a group of anti-diabetic tablets that lower the blood glucose levels. They increase the uptake of glucose by the muscle, reduce the absorption of glucose by the intestine, and reduce the amount of glucose produced by the liver.

Blood glucose monitoring : system of measuring blood glucose levels at home, using special reagent sticks or a special meter.

Blood sugar : the level of glucose in the blood.

Brittle diabetes : term used to describe a type of diabetes that varies from good control to poor control, and shows great fluctuations of sugar levels daily.

Calorie : a unit of measurement by means of which the amount of energy produced in the human body by different kinds of foods is calculated. A calorie is the amount of heat needed to raise the temperature of 1 gramme of water by 1^0 C. In medicine, energy contents of food are expressed in kilocalories (kcals). One kilocalorie is equal to 1,000 calories.

Carbohydrates : one of the three main constituents of food (the other two are protein and fat). They are one of the main sources of calories in food; they supply the energy used in moving, working or just breathing. Composing mainly starches and sugars, they provide 4 calories per gramme.

Cardiovascular : relating to the system through which blood circulates, consisting of the heart, arteries, capillaries and veins.

Cholesterol : a substance present in the blood, the brain, and all other tissues throughout the body, as well as in many food. Chemically it is a steroid. Excess cholesterol in the blood will stick to artery walls, clogging them, thereby leading to atheroscelerosis.

Clear insulin : soluble or regular insulin.

Cloudy insulin : longer-acting insulin with fine particles of protamine or zinc.

Coma : a state of deep unconsciousness from which a person cannot be wakened. Too much or too little insulin in cases of diabetes may also result in coma. The brain stops operating in its normal way, and the patient no longer reacts intelligently to stimuli.

Complications : long-term consequences of imperfectly controlled diabetes.

Control : generally refers to blood glucose control. The objective of good control is to achieve normal blood glucose levels.

Dehydration : abnormal loss of fluid from the body. Water makes up the greater part of the blood and the protoplasm, the fundamental material of which the body is composed. In dehydration, thirst is extreme, the mouth is dry and the skin is doughy and unresilient, urine is dark; and the patient becomes lethargic, with nausea developing.

Dextrose : the commercial name for glucose.

Diabetes insipidus : this rare disease has nothing in common with diabetes mellitus, except the persistent passing of large volumes of urine and constant thirst. A disturbance of vasopressin, a secretion of the pituitary glands, which controls the rate at which water is removed from the kidneys, causes it.

Diabetes mellitus : a disorder of the pancreas characterised by a high glucose level. This develops due to the body's inability to make proper use of ingested food as a result of insufficient availability of insulin.

Diabetic coma : extreme form of hyperglycaemia, usually with keto-acidosis, causing unconsciousness.

Diuretics : a substance that increases the output of urine by the kidneys.

Edema (Oedema) : an abnormal accumulation of fluid in body cavities or tissues, producing swelling.

Enzyme : a catalyst produced by living cells, which helps to speed up biological processes. They control chemical changes, in which complex substances are broken down into forms in which they may be used by the body.

Exchanges : portions of carbohydrate foods in the diabetes diet which can be exchanged for another. 1 exchange = 10 gm carbohydrate.

Fat : a type of food and one of the essential elements in the diet. Fats supply energy in concentrated form.

Fibre : dietary fibre is part of vegetables and grains that is not broken down by digestive juices in the intestine. It holds water in the intestine, adds bulk to stools, and softens them.

Free foods : foods which contain so little carbohydrate and very little or no calories that diabetics may have liberal helpings of them without counting them in their diet.

Fructose : a natural sugar found in fruit and honey. Since it does not require insulin for its metabolism, it is often used as a sweetener in diabetic foods.

Gangrene : the death of tissues caused by lack of oxygen in the cells, usually the result of the blood supply being cut off.

Gestational diabetes : diabetes occurring during pregnancy.

Glucagon : a hormone produced by the alpha cells in the pancreas which causes a rise in blood glucose by freeing glycogen from the liver.

Glucose : form of sugar made by digestion of carbohydrates. It causes a rapid rise in the blood sugar, or blood glucose level. All starches finally break down into glucose, as do all sugars.

Glucose tolerance test : a test used in the diagnosis of diabetes. The patient eats sugar in the form of glucose. At about half-hourly intervals, the urine and blood are examined to discover the amount of sugar present. The results show how the body is using the sugar.

Glycaemia : the normal presence of sugar (glucose) in the bloodstream. Too much sugar in the blood is called hyperglycaemia, and too little is called hypoglycaemia.

Glycogen : a form of starch in which energy-producing glucose is stored in the liver and muscles.

Glycosuria : the present of a large quantity of sugar in the urine.

Glycosylated haemoglobin : another name for haemoglobin A_1.

Haemoglobin A_1 : the part of haemoglobin of red blood cell which has glucose attached to it.

Honeymoon period : time when the dose of insulin drops shortly after starting insulin treatment. It lasts for a short period.

Hormone : any of the several substances present in very small amounts in the blood and producing specific effects in the body.

Hyperglycaemia : a condition in which a person has too much sugar (glucose) in his blood, generally because his pancreas is not producing enough insulin.

Hypoglycaemia : any abnormally low level of glucose in the blood, generally due to an excess of insulin.

Insulin : the hormone produced by the pancreas, in particular by the cell groups on the pancreas known as the islets of Langerhans. It controls the process by which glucose in the blood is converted into energy.

Islets of Langerhans : clusters of cells scattered through the tissues of the pancreas, which produce the hormone, insulin.

Juvenile diabetes : insulin-dependent diabetes. So called because most patients receiving insulin develop diabetes under the age of 40.

Ketoacidosis : poor diabetic control in which ketone bodies that are toxic build up in the blood and cause it to become acidic. It may induce diabetic coma.

Ketones : acid substances formed when body fat is used up to provide energy.

Ketonuria : presence of ketones in the urine.

Lactose : a combination of glucose and galactose, also known as milk sugar.

Maturity onset diabetes : another term for non-insulin-dependent diabetes, commonly occurring in people who are middle-aged and overweight.

Metabolism : all the processes, changes and chemical reactions that occur in the body in order to maintain life. It involves converting food into body tissues – building it into living flesh, blood and bone.

Nephropathy : kidney damage in which the kidney becomes so leaky that albumin appears in the urine.

Neuropathy : damage to the nerves which may be peripheral or autonomic.

Pancreas : a dual purpose gland, lying across and behind the stomach. It produces the pancreatic juice needed for digestion, and insulin and glucagons that control the way the body uses sugar.

Peripheral neuropathy : damage to the nerves supplying the muscles and skin, leading to numbness.

Polydipsia : being excessively thirsty and drinking to much, sign of untreated diabetes.

Polyuria : passing of large amounts of urine due to excess glucose from the bloodstream.

Protein : a complex chemical compound that forms an essential part of every living cell. They make up part of chromosomes, enzymes, blood plasma and haemoglobin. They contain nitrogen, carbon, hydrogen and oxygen, and other elements.

Pyelonephritis : a serious condition in which the initial infection has spread from the urine-collecting part of the kidney into adjacent parts.

Renal threshold : the level of glucose in the blood above which it will begin to spill into the urine.

Retina : the light-sensitive area at the back of the eye.

Retinopathy : damage to the retina in the eye.

Saccharin : an intensely sweet, white, crystalline compound derived from coal tar and petroleum, and used as a substitute for sugar.

Sorbitol : a sugar alcohol that is absorbed by the body more slowly than glucose. It usually causes no significant effect upon the blood sugar level but has the same number of calories as ordinary sugar.

Steroids : a general term for any of a large group of naturally occurring substances with a similar kind of chemical structure, many of which play important roles in the body.

Sucrose : a natural sugar derived from sugarcane or sugar beet. It has a high carbohydrate and calorie content.

Toxaemia : the medical term for the presence of any poisonous substance in the circulating blood, the condition commonly known as blood poisoning.

Vascular : a term that refers to the blood vessels.

Vitamins : a group of substances found in small amounts in most foods. They are essential for well-balanced diet.

• • •